MW01234486

Recipe 4 Success

R4S

HE + E + MBC = R4S

Your solution to achieving sustainable weight loss, attaining weight mastery, and remaining healthy for life

Dr. Firlande Volcy

Recipe 4 Success
R4S
HE + E + MBC = R4S

Your solution to achieving sustainable weight loss, attaining weight mastery, and remaining healthy for life.

Dr. Firlande Volcy

First Edition – June 2016
ISBN-13: 978-1534626898
ISBN-10: 1534626891

Disclaimer: This book is solely for informational and educational purposes. It is not intended to replace or supersede medical advice. Consult your healthcare professional if you have questions about your health.

Exercise photograph courtesy of Martine Volcy / Zhengathemodel

To all seeking knowledge.

Table of Contents

Acknowledgements

I wish to express my gratitude towards everyone in my close circle of family and friends who have helped and supported me directly and indirectly in writing this book. Thank you to those who came before me and imparted the knowledge necessary to solidify my thoughts. I am forever indebted to all the people who have crossed my path and have ultimately contributed to this project.

Thank you, Dr. Firlande Volcy

Introduction

Humankind has been searching for "the" solution to weight loss for decades and many have devised diet plans, ideas, and responses to what they perceive as being the solution to sustainable weight loss. Ultimately, we all have the answer within our fingertips. It's not rocket science, it's not a magic pill, it's not a quick weight loss scam. We are well aware that healthy eating and exercise are the main elements indispensable to sustainable weight loss. However, there's one crucial component, often disregarded, that bridges the gap and accelerates the process, **the mind-body connection**.

> **Healthy Eating (HE)**
> **Exercise (E)**
> **Mind-Body Connection (MBC)**

Healthy eating, exercise, and mind-body connection are your combined solution to achieving sustainable weight loss, attaining weight mastery, and remaining healthy for life. When those three components are utilized efficiently and simultaneously, you have a true **Recipe 4 Success (R4S)**.

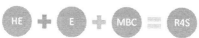

Undoubtedly, other factors may affect weight gain, including hormonal imbalances, stress, unhappiness, eating disorders, steroid intake, etc. Nevertheless, once those conditions are resolved or ruled out, MBC combined with HE and E will yield immediate weight loss success.

What makes this book different from all the other weight loss books out there?

R4S is not your typical weight loss book. It travels beyond weight loss to deliver all the necessary information and tools to help anyone succeed in their health and wellness journey and conquer weight.

- Most people who embark in weight loss programs fail because they lack the basic concept and required knowledge of the components and nutrients in the foods they ingest daily. **Part I** provides a complete breakdown of those components and nutrients (i.e., carbohydrates, proteins, fats, vitamins, minerals, and phytochemicals) and their implications and significance in supporting health and wellness.

- **Part II** introduces a whole foods guide and perfectly groups the nutrients into their individual food categories to ease the selection process. In addition, Part II establishes the most beneficial methods to utilize foods as nourishment including proper food shopping, preparing and cooking, combining, and eating.

- **Part III** refines the importance of physical activity, describes the various types of exercises, and proposes a comprehensive exercise training program to take the guesswork out of your workout.

- Finally, **Part IV** bridges the gap between healthy eating and exercise with the mind-body connection. You are provided with superior strategies such as meditation, positive affirmation, visualization, self-love, and journaling to aid in the achievement of balance and homeostasis and accelerate weight loss.

A comprehensive, step-by-step, and easy to uphold 9-week program immediately follows and is divided into 3 phases with each phase lasting 21 days:

Phase I – Detox Phase

Phase II – Fat Burning Phase

Phase III – Weight Mastery / Healthy 4 Life Phase

Phase I is detoxification phase. You will remove junk (toxins, fats, and mucus) out of your body to boost your immune system, jumpstart weight loss, and prepare for fat burning phase. The diet will be light, expanding, and uplifting to support the body in cleansing. The exercise will be easy to avoid early burnout and injury.

Phase II is all about maximizing on fat loss. In this phase, you are taught to utilize fat metabolism as fuel rather than carbohydrates. This process will upsurge fat loss by tapping into fat reserved while preserving muscle mass. The diet will be devoid of starches and heavy fatty foods to facilitate fat mobilization and metabolism. The exercise shifts from walking to interval training to increase physical fitness and burn the most calories.

Phase III is about implementing and incorporating what you've learned in the previous sections to acquire weight mastery and remain healthy for life. The diet reflects how you should eat beyond the program to maintain a healthy weight. The exercises vary to suit your body type and schedule.

Each phase is designed to prepare your body for success in the subsequent phase. For instance, the first phase cleanses the body of toxins to allow fat mobilization and excretion in the next phase more efficient. Once you've grasped how to mobilize fats, you will eat accordingly in the last phase to achieve weight mastery.

Furthermore, each phase contains:

1) Daily meal plans that combine healthy choices with the adequate amount of calories and portion size to aid weight loss and avoid starvation.
2) An extensive exercise program to increase physical fitness and endurance.
3) A mind-body component to improve mental fitness and stability.
4) Three 21-day challenges, which target all the components of R4S, healthy eating, exercise, and mind-body connection.

Easy to follow recipes and tips for sustainable weight loss conclude this well designed and comprehensive health book.

There are no quick fixes and no short cuts to achieving sustainable weight loss. You have to do the work. The bulk of the work is done for you. Your only task is to follow the program as outlined. By combining the mind-body connection with healthy eating and exercise, you can accelerate weight loss and achieve weight mastery in a timely manner. Remember, you are giving up a little to gain a lot, so give it your all and your efforts will be rewarding. Stick with it for the duration of the program and when you fall off just get back on. Be patient with yourself and enjoy the process!!!

R4S is your guide to better health, improvement of physical fitness, and development of inner strength and a positive mental attitude.

HE + E + MBC = R4S

Part I

Components and Nutrients in Foods

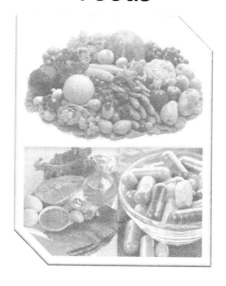

❀ ❀ ❀

"Let thy food be thy medicine and medicine thy food"
Thomas Jefferson

Food is medicine and when utilized wholesomely, it will manage, treat, and even cure many preventable illnesses especially obesity, diabetes, and hypertension. Thus, to commence any health regimen or weight loss program it is imperative to acquire knowledge on the basic components and nutrients in foods. Subsequently, that knowledge will guide you towards better food choices beyond the limitation of the program.

Food provides the #1 source of key essential nutrients like **water, carbohydrates, fats, proteins, minerals, and vitamins** to sustain life and health. Those nutrients are frequently grouped into two main categories **macronutrients** and **micronutrients**. Each type of nutrient has specific functions yet works collectively and synergistically to maintain health and support the body in carrying out its proper function.

In the next few sections, you will learn about macronutrients, micronutrients, phytochemicals, and some supplements that aid in weight loss.

Macronutrients

Water
Carbohydrates
Protein
Fat

Macronutrients are the nutrients that the body needs in larger quantities. They are the elementary building blocks of a complete and balanced diet. They generate energy, nourish the body, and have various other functions. Understanding their importance and the roles they play in weight loss and health will yield success.

Macronutrients are broken down into four basic nutrients:

1. Water
2. Carbohydrates
3. Fats
4. Proteins

1

Water

"Follow my rule of 10"

2/3rds of the body is comprised of water, making it the most essential nutrient in the body.

What's the importance of water?

Water is the basis of all body fluids including blood, urine, lymph, digestive juices, and perspiration. All cells and organs depend on it to function properly and effectively.

For instance, water:

- ◆ Provides a fluid medium for all chemical reactions in the body to occur,
- ◆ Aids in transport of nutrients into the cells and waste products (e.g., toxins) out of the cells,
- ◆ Is essential for proper circulation, digestion, absorption, and excretion,
- ◆ Regulates the body's temperature, and
- ◆ Helps with weight loss

Too little water intake may result in dehydration (esp. in the summer) and prolong dehydration can cause organ failure. Excessive water consumption can lead to the rare case of water toxicity.

Where can you obtain water?

Since water is one the most abundant nutrient in nature, you have many options. You can choose from natural springs, tap, bottled, well, and many other sources. The key is to consume pure, clean, and *alkaline water to ensure the body's proper function, maintain health, and lose weight. You can also obtain water indirectly from foods or from metabolism, as a by-product, but you need to make up the balance by drinking an adequate amount each day.

To check the pH of your drinking water, purchase a pH test strip at your nearest pharmacy and test your water. A pH of 8 or above, will keep your body alkaline and your organs well hydrated.

Let's break it down!!!

How much water should you be drinking?

Your body requires an adequate amount of water per day to lose weight and preserve health. Hence, **water must be your #1 nutrient**. Occasionally, dehydration is the leading cause of overeating and obesity especially in the summer because it is frequently confused with hunger. People tend to increase food consumption rather than water intake.

Increasing daily water intake will:

- Allow better flow and circulation,
- Reduce inflammation and appetite,
- Keep your organs hydrated,
- Accelerate fat loss,
- Rid the body of toxins,
- Decrease cravings,
- Shrink fat cells,
- Decrease weight gain, and
- Combat hunger by keeping you full longer.

Water should be your *best ally*. It is indispensable to life and to weight loss. I recommend a gallon of water per day or half your body weight in ounces. For instance, if you weigh 160lbs divide that by 2. Your daily minimum water intake would be about 80 ounces.

160lbs/2 = 80 oz. of water

If you engage in strenuous physical activities and/or work in the sun, double your water intake and/or add electrolytes to the water to 1) replace water and mineral lost and 2) stay hydrated.

*In the first phase of the program, you have a **water challenge.** Your goal is to steadily increase your water intake until you reach a gallon on day 21 (assuming you're drinking less than that amount). If you already drink an adequate amount of water per day but never quite reach a gallon, start from where you are and increase by 4-8 ounces each day.*

Infused Water

Water infusion is the process of extracting chemical compounds, flavors, and colors from plant materials into the water. I highly recommend infused water daily because of the following benefits, infused water:

- Increases alkalinity,
- Increases diuresis,
- Aids in weight loss,
- Cleanses the urinary track,
- Clears the skin, and
- Quenches thirst rapidly

You can infuse your water with fruits, vegetables, and/or herbs. My favorites are lemon, cucumber, pineapple, and mint leaves infused water. Increase cucumber and watermelon infused water consumption in summer to remain hydrated.

Drinking water during meals

Drinking water or any other fluids during meals is highly discouraged because the excess water can dilute the enzymes necessary for digestion rendering them less viable. This may lead to indigestion, nutrient malabsorption, heartburn, leaky gut, and irritable bowel. I suggest allowing a small window of 10-30 minutes before and after your meal to drink water. This will enable your own natural digestive juices to begin assimilation.

Moreover, proper mastication, which increases saliva, provides ample liquid for a smooth descend to the esophagus into the stomach and more fluid is unwarranted. However, for those who must have water during meals, I devised a **rule of 10** to facilitate with the process.

Drink 10 ounces of water 10 minutes before and 10 minutes after your meals.

♦ **10 minutes before**:

Drinking 10 ounces of water 10 minutes before your meal will quench any thirst, clean your palate, and deter overeating due to dehydration.

♦ **10 minutes after**:

Delaying by at least 10 minutes after may prevent enzyme dilution. In addition, make it a hobbit to drink regularly 10-30 minutes after meals to fill your belly, deter overeating, and facilitate communication between your brain and stomach.

Remember, to reach your daily water goal of a minimum of half your body weight in ounces, you must drink water in between meals as well.

What will you need for the program?

♦ *An excellent water filter, if you are drinking tap water, preferably an alkaline filter that will get rid of impurities in the water while simultaneously change the pH from acidic to alkaline.*

◆ *A 32 ounces or larger plastic (BPH free) or glass water bottle to carry with you at all times.*

◆ *A gallon-size pitcher, water dispenser, or infuser bottle for water infusion.*

2

Carbohydrates

"Count your Carbs"

Carbohydrate (aka carbs) is the body's primary source of energy. It is the energy from the sun captured by plants, algae, and some bacteria during photosynthesis.

What's the importance of carbohydrates in the diet?

Carbohydrates provide rapid energy to sustain life. In fact, glucose, a type of carbohydrate, is the principal source of energy utilized by the brain and red blood cells. In prolong state of starvation or famine, the body breaks down fats into glucose to feed the brain. In the 2nd phase of the program, we will force the body into utilizing its stored fats as fuel to promote lipolysis by keeping carbs at a minimal in the diet.

Most people in North America fall victim to excessive consumption of carbs, which can lead to obesity, malnutrition with farinaceous dystrophy in children. Higher amount of carbs are necessary during strenuous physical activity to feed the brain and for proper growth in children.

A deficiency of carbohydrates is rare but when it happens, (e.g., high protein diet) it can cause ketosis, mineral loss, and dehydration.

Where are your carbs?

Carbs are found in abundance in plant foods such as vegetables, fruits, grains, peas, and legumes and in some animal products like milk and milk goods. Fortunately, not all carbs are created equal. Some carbs are higher in sugar and starch, which tend to increase blood sugar levels and others are higher in fiber and water, which balance blood sugar levels. You need more of the latter in the diet and less of the former.

Groups of Carbohydrates:

Carbs are classified into monosaccharides, disaccharides, oligosaccharides, and polysaccharides.

1. Monosaccharides

Monosaccharides or **"simple sugars"** contain one sugar molecule and cannot be broken down into smaller or simpler compounds. They arise in nature (e.g., honey or fruit sugar) or as intermediate products of digestion (e.g., break down of grains).

Types of Monosaccharides:

- **Glucose**: is the main source of energy for the brain and red blood cells. It is the most abundant sugar in nature.
- **Fructose**: sweetest sugar, readily converted to fat or glucose. Found in fruits, honey, corn syrup, and molasses.
- **Galactose**: only found with glucose as lactose (i.e. milk sugar).

2. Disaccharides

Disaccharides are also "simple sugars" since they contain only two sugar molecules linked together by glycosidic bonds.

Types of Disaccharides:

- **Sucrose** = glucose + fructose: found in table sugar and naturally in fruits and vegetables.
- **Maltose** = glucose + glucose: found in sprouting plants; used in beverages such as beer brewing.

♦ **Lactose** = glucose + galactose: milk sugar – found in milk and milk products.

3. Oligosaccharides

Oligosaccharides contain short chains of simple sugars (3-10) linked together. They serve as prebiotics in the diet and are frequently added to commercial foods as sweeteners or fibers. Some common types of oligosaccharides include:

♦ **Fructo-oligosaccharides (FOS)** found in Jerusalem artichokes, onions, and canned foods.

♦ **Galacto-oligosaccharides (GOS)** found in beans, peas, lentils, cabbages, and whole grains.

4. Polysaccharides

Polysaccharides or "**complex carbs**" contain long chain of sugar molecules. The common types of complex carbohydrates include starch, glycogen, and fiber.

♦ **Starch** is the most common storage form of polysaccharides found in plants. When ingested, it is broken down to simple sugars and utilized by the body for energy. Grains, legumes, cereals, potatoes, and peas are all examples of starches.

♦ **Glycogen** is the main storage form of glucose found in animal cells like the liver and skeletal muscle. It is not found in food.

♦ **Fiber** is the major component of plant cell walls. Diets low in fiber can lead to arteriosclerosis, diverticulosis, constipation, and have greater risks of cancer especially colon cancer. Supplemental fiber taken in excessive amount may reduce the absorption of zinc, iron, and other minerals and may cause constipation.

More on Fiber:

There are two types of fiber 1) **soluble** and 2) **insoluble** fibers.

♦ **Soluble fibers**: are partially digested by bacteria then absorbed in the large intestine. They increase stool bulk by absorbing water while speeding movement of food through the digestive track. When they absorb water, they turn into gel-like goo (e.g., oatmeal).

- **Insoluble fibers**: are mostly indigestible by the body's digestive enzymes and intestinal bacteria. They don't absorb water and when consumed in excess, they can irritate the intestinal lining causing colitis. They are found in seeds, fruit skins, celery, whole grains, etc.

Benefits of fiber

Having enough fiber in the diet is important to health and weight loss. Fiber has many health benefits. Fiber,

- Keeps the bowel clean, thereby increasing the amount of calories you excrete out of the colon.
- Delays the rate by which the stomach empties.
- Improves sugar tolerance (great for diabetics)
- Increases the amount of chewing.
- Keeps you full longer.
- Decreases appetite.
- Decreases cholesterol levels.

Soluble Fibers	
Hemicellulose: plant cell walls, oat, gum, bran	**Gums**: oatmeal and dried beans
Mucilage: fenugreek seed, peas, psyllium seed, and flax seed	**Pectin**: apples, pears, citrus rind, beans, cabbage, whole grains, and root vegetables
Insoluble Fibers	
Lignan: flax seeds, sesame seed, rye, wheat, oat, barley, and soybeans	**Cellulose**: whole grains, bran, cabbage, peas, beans, celery, root vegetables, and fruit skins

Let's break it down!!!

How much carbs do you need to consume per day?

The amount of carbs you consume per day will determine overall success – weight loss or weight gain. More carbs in the diet will cause weight gain when not accompany by exercise and less carbs will push your body towards fat metabolism as fuel.

The amount of carbs will differ with each phase of the program.

> **Phase I:** 100-120g per day (80% leafy and non-starchy, 5% starches, & 15% fruits)
>
> **Phase II:** 60-70g per day (99% leafy and non-starchy vegetables, 1% fruits)
>
> **Phase III:** 100-150g per day until you reach weight mastery (80% leafy and non-starchy, 20% starches & fruits)

Why do you need to maintain your carbs at a minimum?

Carbohydrates provide energy and when they are not utilized for that purpose, your body stores them as fats in the form of triglycerides. For instance, when you ingest a potato:

- It is broken down into mostly simple sugars like glucose and perhaps fiber if you eat the skin.
- The sugar travels to the blood stream to feed the brain or the muscles during exercise.
- Excess sugars are picked up and carried out of the bloodstream by insulin. They are then stored by glucagon in the cells (liver and muscle cells) via a process called glycogenesis for later use.
- Consistent amounts of sugar, which the body has no use for, is stored as fat via lipogenesis.

Meanwhile since your goal is weight loss / fat loss, decreasing your daily carbs intake will allow your body to tap into its reserved fats, break them down, and utilize them as fuel. The low carb diet, which is comprised of mostly fiber, will add bulk and nutrients, decrease appetite, and assist with satiety.

What will you need for the program?

- *A food scale for weighing fruits and vegetables*
- *Salad spinner to remove extra water out of leafy green vegetables*
- *Mason jar and a mesh lid for sprouting grains and legumes*
- *Mearing cups*

3

Proteins

"Keep your Protein Lean & Clean"

Proteins are the most abundant macromolecules in living cells in the body next to water. They are comprised of amino acids, the building blocks of all proteins.

Why are proteins important?

They are the basic materials of life and are necessary for blood clotting, acid/alkaline balance in blood, and the formation of enzymes, hormones, antibodies, hair, nails, and the lens protein of the eye. You need protein to keep your body functioning properly and to maintain muscles, bones, organs, and other tissues.

Whenever the body makes a protein, (e.g., for muscle building) it needs a variety of amino acids both from dietary protein (essential) and from the body's own pool of amino acids (nonessential). Chronic shortage of amino acids, which can occur with vegetarian when the diet lacks essential amino acids, cease the production of protein and can lead to weakness, apathy, immune depression (low disease resistance), edema, and liver failure. Dietary protein in excess can result in renal and rheumatic disease, gout, and acidification of the blood since proteins require an acidic pH for digestion.

Classification of amino acids:

1) **Essential**: cannot be synthesized by the body and must be supplied by the diet.
2) **Non-essential**: synthesized by substances in the body and do not need to be supplemented in the diet.
3) **Conditional**: they are nonessential amino acids that only need to be supplied by the diet in times of illness and stress.

Amino Acids		
Essential	**Nonessential**	**Conditional**
Histidine	Alanine	Arginine
Isoleucine	Asparagine	Cysteine
Leucine	Aspartate	Glutamine
Lysine	Glutamate	Glycine
Methionine		Ornithine
Phenylalanine		Proline
Threonine		Serine
Tryptophan		
Valine		

Dietary proteins are categorized into two groups since both plant and animal foods supply extensive amount of proteins but in dissimilar amounts:

1) Complete proteins:

Provide all nine essential amino acids that the body needs. All animal products provide complete proteins. Soybeans are one of the most complete vegetable protein source, missing only one essential amino acid, methionine.

13

2) **Incomplete proteins:**

Most plants provide incomplete proteins. They only contain some of the essential amino acids and need to be combined to form complete proteins. For example, combining rice and beans would make a complete protein.

Benefits of dietary protein:

- Increases lean muscle mass.
- Decreases the rate of gastric emptying, which keeps you full longer.
- Repairs muscle tissues following exercise.
- Increases weight loss and weight maintenance.

Let's break it down!!!

How much protein is necessary in the diet to help you reach your goal weight?

Protein is your **second best ally** (water is 1st).

You need an adequate amount of protein in the diet since protein is thermic in nature. It has much lower available calories for the body to use and store as fat compare to carbs. Meaning, when you ingest protein, it is broken down into its building block to produce muscles rather than glucose for energy. Protein can also increase your metabolic rate by as much as 30%. Body builders increase muscle mass by consuming high amounts of protein from both animal and plant sources.

If you are a vegetarian, you can obtain just as much protein from vegetables, nuts, and grains. Sprouting nuts, grains, and beans increase the available protein content and digestibility. Food combining will play a key role in assuring a well-balanced diet. For example, combining sprouted grains with sprouted legumes can provide excellent source of protein.

The amount of protein you ingest differs in each phase. You consume the most protein in the fat burning phase to allow fat break down and less in the detox phase to support the liver. The amount normalizes in the last phase.

Phase I: 3-4 ounces of lean protein per meal

Phase II: 4-6 ounces of lean protein per meal

Phase III: 3-5 ounces of lean protein per meal

Caution: High consumption of protein (10oz or more per meal) has been linked to gout. Follow the program to avoid overconsumption.

What will you need for the program?

♦ *A small grill or grill pan for easy grilling and faster meals*

♦ *Food Thermometer*

♦ *A food scale – to weigh cooked animal proteins*

4

Fats

"Are Fats Good for you?"

Fats are essential for the proper functioning of the body.

♦ They facilitate transport of fat soluble vitamins (A, D, E, and K).

♦ They can serve as pigments for the retina (vitamin A), cofactors (vitamin K), detergents (bile salts), transporters, hormones (sex hormones) and anchors for membrane proteins.

♦ Fats or lipids are insoluble in water.

They are categorized by:

1) Fatty acids and oils: the principal storage forms of energy in many organisms

2) **Lipids and steroids**: make up the biological membranes. The fats present in all foods are composed of triglycerides (96-98%), which are simple lipids made of glycerin and fatty acids.

Types of fatty acids:
1. **Saturated Fats:** (aka "bad" fats)
   - Tend to increase LDL blood cholesterol levels
   - Usually solid at room temperature
   - Mostly found in animal products (dairy, meat, margarine, lard)
   - Found in some vegetable oils: coconut oil, palm kernel oil, vegetable shortening
2. **Monounsaturated Fats**: (aka "good" fats)
   - Tend to reduce LDLs level without affecting HDLs
   - Mostly plant based, found in vegetable and nut oils such as olive, peanut, and canola oils
3. **Polyunsaturated Fats**: (better fats)
   - Tend to lower LDLs and increase HDLs cholesterol levels
   - Should not be heated.
   - Mostly found in vegetable products such as soybean, safflower, flax, and sunflower oils.
   - They contain substances beneficial to health such as lecithin, phytosterols, and vitamin E.
4. **Essential fatty acids:**
   - "Essential" fatty acids (EFA) are fatty acids that must be supplied by the diet.
   - Examples: linoleic, linolenic, and arachidonic acid.
   - Most polyunsaturated fats contain essential fatty acids.

Let's break it Down!!!

How much fat do you really need in the diet?

Your body produces its own fat, but an adequate amount is required from the diet to maintain health. Your daily fat intake percentage will defer with each phase.

Phase I: comprise about 15-20% of daily intake

Phase II: increase to 60% of daily caloric intake

Phase III: about 20% of daily caloric intake

In phase III, fats are at a higher percentage to allow the body to burn fat more efficiently. Fats are naturally high in calories, by increasing the total amount of fats even slightly; the percentage also increases. For example, 1 tbsp. of olive oil is approximately 119 calories. 1 ounce of cheese equates to 110 calories (dairy products such as milk and cheese are high in fats unless the fat is removed). When added to the total daily caloric intake, you've already consumed 229 calories.

Beware of the types of fats you consume. Too much saturated fats in the diet can clog your arteries and cause cardiovascular diseases. Add more polyunsaturated fats, which can improve cardiovascular health and prevent hypercholesterolemia. (See Part II for a list of good and bad fats.)

Micronutrients

Vitamins

Minerals

Micronutrients serve as regulators intervening in various processes and functions of the body. They are called micronutrients because the body needs them in a much smaller quantity for survival. Nonetheless, they play key roles in keeping the body healthy by supporting the immune system, the reproductive organs, the bones, and the heart. They include:

1. **Vitamins**
   - Fat Soluble Vitamins
   - Water Soluble Vitamins
2. **Minerals**
   - Macrominerals
   - Microminerals

1
Vitamins

Vitamins are organic substances required in the diet in smaller quantities for the body to function properly. They are obtained primarily from ingestion of foods. They serve many functions and are essential to life. They are categorized into **fat-soluble** and **water-soluble** vitamins.

Fat Soluble Vitamins
Characteristics:
   - They are soluble in oil or fatty solutions.
   - They are absorbed in the small intestine with the help of bile salts and juices from the pancreatic organ and stored in the liver and fat cells.
   - They may take days to be excreted out of the body as compared to water-soluble vitamins, which are excreted within a few hours.

♦ They play essential roles in a variety of critical biological processes such as vision, maintenance of bones, and blood coagulation.

Fat-soluble	Functions	Sources
Vitamin A	Powerful antioxidant – major role in day and night vision, reproduction, bone growth and maturation, renewal of skin and mucous membranes, and immune health.	Organ meats, butter, eggs, fish liver oils, chicken, beans, peas, peppers, green, yellow and orange vegetables and fruits
Vitamin D	Essential for normal growth and development, bone health, absorption and metabolism of calcium, phosphorus, and magnesium	The sun, fish, liver, animal flesh, dairy, eggs, fortified cereals and breads
Vitamin E	Powerful antioxidant, anti-inflammatory & anticoagulant; important for skin, muscle, heart, brain, and reproductive health	Plant oils, organ meats, fish, nuts, seeds, wheat germ, avocado, eggs, butter
Vitamin K	Necessary for normal blood clotting, bone formation and repair; aid in the conversion of glucose to glycogen for storage in the liver	K1: leafy green vegetables, broccoli, brussel sprouts, asparagus, cabbages, alfalfa; K2: organ meats, milk, eggs, and cheese

Water Soluble Vitamins
Characteristics:

♦ They are soluble in water solutions.

♦ They are components or precursors of important biological substances known as coenzymes.

♦ They must be replenished frequently and must be taken in daily, as they can only be stored for a few hours in tissues before they are excreted out of the body.

- They may be lost when foods are overcooked and improperly handled and stored.

Water-Soluble	Functions	Food Sources
B1 **Thiamine**	Essential for growth, normal appetite, digestion, and healthy nerves	Brewer's yeast, organ meats, wheat germ, seeds, nuts, beans, rice, oatmeal, millet, potatoes, pork
B2 **Riboflavin**	Prevents fissures at corners of mouth; alleviates eye irritation and photophobia	Brewer's yeast, organ meats, red meat, poultry, almonds, wheat germ, grains, mushrooms, eggs, peppers, vegetables
B3 **Niacin**	Lowers blood cholesterol levels	Brewer's yeast, rice, meat, poultry, fish, nuts, peas, seeds, legumes, milk, eggs, grains
B5 **Pantothenic Acid**	Aids in production of steroid hormones by the adrenal glands	Brewer's yeast, organ meats, mushrooms, avocado, grains, dairy, vegetables, legumes
B6 **Pyridoxine**	Necessary for normal brain function and synthesis of amino acids and hormones	Brewer's yeast, organ meats, sunflower seeds, wheat germ, cold water fish, beans, walnuts, vegetables, nuts, avocado
B12 **Cobalamin**	Needs intrinsic factor to be absorbed; increases energy	Meat, poultry, fish, shellfish, eggs
Biotin	Lowers insulin resistance	Beans, grains, bran, egg yolk, peanuts, pecans, oats
Folic Acid	Prevents neural tube defects in newborns	Brewer's yeast, rice germ, beans, bran, green vegetables, nuts, oats, dates, grains
Vitamin C	Powerful antioxidant; aids in collagen, immune, and soft tissue health, iron absorption and cholesterol excretion	peppers, guavas, leafy vegetables, broccoli, cauliflower, red cabbage, berries, citrus fruits, mangos, onions, peas, squash

General Functions of B Vitamins:

B vitamins function as cellular metabolism and/or energy production. They aid in amino acids conversions, metabolism of carbohydrates, proteins, fats, and nucleic acids, formation of red blood cell (RBC), and maintenance of nerve conductions. They increase overall energy.

2
Minerals

Minerals are inorganic compounds (containing no carbon), vital for biological and physiological processes in the body. They provide structure to the skeletal system, regulate water and acid-base balance in the body, and promote nerve impulses. Through erosion, they are carried into the soil, groundwater, and sea then taken up by plants and later consumed by animals and humans. There are many minerals found in the body but only a few are considered essential.

Minerals are categorized into two categories:

- Macrominerals
- Microminerals

Macrominerals: found in abundance in the body and are necessary for the body's proper function. The well researched macrominerals include:

- **Calcium**: 99% is found in bones and teeth
- **Chloride**: mostly found in the extracellular fluids
- **Magnesium**: 55-60% are found in bones, 20-25% in muscles, and the rest in soft tissues and extracellular fluids
- **Phosphorus**: 85% found in bones, 14% in soft tissues, and 1% in blood and body fluids.

- **Potassium**: 98% of potassium is found in intracellular fluid
- **Sodium**: 70% of sodium is found in extracellular fluid of nerve and muscle tissue and 30% on surface of bone crystals.

Minerals	Functions	Sources
Calcium	Aids in mineralization of bone, blood clotting, enzyme regulation, nerve conduction, muscle contraction, and membrane permeability	Broccoli, dairy products, dried fruits, leafy greens, tofu, sardines, salmon, kelp, dulse, wheat germ, miso, Brazil nuts, grains, seeds.
Chloride	Maintains the body's fluid and acid-base balance, major secretory electrolyte in the GI tract (for gastric juices)	Table salt as sodium chloride
Magnesium	Involves in protein synthesis energy production, bone growth, nerves, and muscles function, and regulation of normal heart beat	Nuts, seeds, legumes, whole-grain cereals, fruits, chlorophyll in green leafy vegetables
Phosphorus	Plays vital role in energy metabolism, bones and teeth structure	Meat, poultry, fish, eggs, milk and dairy products, nuts, legumes, cereals, grains and chocolate
Potassium	Involves in nerve impulses, muscle contraction, healthy hair growth; proper function of the heart and kidneys; prevention of fermentation and autointoxication	Bananas, potatoes (with skin), oranges, dried fruits, meat, poultry, dairy products
Sodium	Helps regulate blood pressure and water balance in the body.	Table salt

Microminerals: found at trace amounts. The most abundant micromineral in the body is Iron and the second most abundant is Zinc.

Minerals	Functions	Sources
Arsenic	Necessary for certain amino acids metabolism and phospholipid synthesis	Shellfish, fish, eggs, milk, meat, fruits, vegetables; highest amounts are found in the skin, hair and nails
Boron	Aids in mental alertness, psychomotor skills, and cognitive processed of attention and memory, and metabolism of triglycerides and other minerals	Fruits, vegetables, nuts, legumes, wine, cider, beer; low in meat and fish
Chromium	Necessary for metabolism of glucose and synthesis of cholesterol, fats, and proteins	Meats (esp. organ meats), grains, cheese, mushrooms, brewer's yeast, tea, beer, and wine
Copper	Along with iron, it helps in formation of red blood cells. Secreted into the GI tract from saliva, gastric, pancreatic and duodenal juices in large amounts.	Organ meats and shellfish, nuts, seeds, legumes, dried fruits, sweet potatoes
Fluoride	Mineralization of teeth and bones; deposited in community drinking water	Infant formulas, dairy foods, cereals and grains, potatoes, leafy greens, toothpastes
Iodine	Necessary for synthesis of thyroid hormones by thyroid gland, increases metabolism, and protects from radiation damage	Seafood, seaweeds, vegetables, meats, dairy foods, fortified foods (salt), iodates in bread (dough improver)
Iron	Most abundant trace mineral; essential for the formation of hemoglobin (blood) and myoglobin (muscle).	Heme (50-60%): meat, fish, poultry Nonheme (40%): plant foods and dairy products

Manganese	Necessary in normal bone growth and synthesis, energy production, and reproduction; recommended in combination with other trace minerals.	Whole grain cereals, dried fruit, nuts, legumes, and leafy vegetables (processing reduce manganese in grains)
Molybdenum	Necessary for Nitrogen metabolism and activation of certain enzymes in the body; supports bone growth and strengthening of the teeth	Meats (esp. organ meats), legumes, cereals, grains, and vegetables
Nickel	Component of many enzyme systems in plants, including redox reactions, gene regulation, and hydrolysis; concentrated in hair, bone, soft tissues, and thyroid and adrenal glands	Nuts, legumes, grains, chocolate, cured meats, and vegetables, low in animal products
Selenium	Vital antioxidant; protects the immune system, maintain healthy organs, aid in iodine metabolism and antibody production	Plants, organ meats, seafood, soil (varied concentrations) Selenium in the soil is dependent on volcanic ash and rainfall
Silicon	Necessary for formation of collagen in bones and connective tissue, healthy nails, hair, and skin, and calcium absorption in the early stages of bone formation	Whole grains, beer, root vegetables (turnips, burdock, rutabagas)
Vanadium	Required for cellular metabolism, growth, reproduction, insulin utilization, and formation of bones and teeth; inhibits cholesterol synthesis	Whole grains, liver, fish, spinach, black pepper, parsley, mushrooms, oysters, shellfish, beer, and wine
Zinc	Necessary for immune health, enzyme activities, DNA replication, taste and smell acuity, carbohydrates	Red meats (esp. organ meats), seafood, whole grains, leafy and root vegetables

	metabolism, cell division, growth, and repair	

Phytochemicals

Phytochemicals aka Phytonutrients are natural, plant-derived nutrients that give fruits and vegetables their color, fragrance, flavor, and tartness. They are non-vitamin, non-mineral components of foods with significant health benefits. They act as a natural defense system for their host plants- protecting the plants from infections, microbial invasions, weather, and sun damage. They are also the part of the plant that will assure its regeneration.

Phytonutrients are powerful antioxidant, anti-inflammatory, anti-aging, and anti-carcinogenic.

List of Phytochemicals:

- Alkaloids: Caffeine, Theobromine, Theophylline
- Anthocyanins: Cyanidin, Malvidin
- Carotenoids: Beta-carotene, Lutein, Lycopene
- Flavanoids: Epicatechin, Hesperidin, Quercetin, Isorhamnetin, Kaempferol, Myricetin, Naringin, Nobiletin, Proanthocyanidins, Rutin, Tangeretin
- Hydroxycinnamic acids: Chicoric acid, Coumarin, Ferulic acid, Scopoletin
- Isoflavones: Daidzein, Genistein
- Lignans: Silymarin
- Monophenols: Hydroxytyrosol
- Monoterpenes: Geraniol, Limonene

- Organosulfides: Allicin, Glutathione, Indole-3-Carbinol, Isothiocyanates, Sulforaphane
- Other phytochemicals: Damnacanthal, Digoxin, Phytic acid
- Phenolic Acids: Capsaicin, Ellagic acid, Gallic Acid, Rosmarinic acid, Tannic acid
- Phytosterols: Beta-Sitosterol
- Saponins
- Stylbenes: Pterostilbene, Resveratrol
- Triterpenoids: Ursolic acid
- Xanthophylls: Astaxanthin, Beta-cryptoxanthin

Supplements

o supplement or not?

If we lived in a world, where everything we consumed, naturally contained all the vitamins, minerals, and phytochemicals we need to sustain health and wellness, then we would not have to supplement. Unfortunately, our soil is depleted and our foods are highly processed, genetically modified, and devoid of any nutritional values. We don't obtain what the body needs from our foods to function optimally.

Weight gain is mainly a problem of malnutrition caused by nutritional deficiency of both macro- and micro- nutrients. I highly recommend supplementations.

Various supplements can aid in maintaining health and wellness; I have only included a few in this book. For additional information on nutritional supplements, purchase a nutrition book or visit any government websites on nutrition.

I listed a few recommendations below you can add to your regimen that will aid in weight loss.

Supplements	Function
Chromium	Decreases sugar cravings
Kelp	Sea vegetable, contains iodine, which increases metabolic rate
EFA	Great for appetite control
CLA	Assists in fat burning and muscle building and retention
Vitamin C	Speeds up metabolism
Vitamin B complex	Increases energy and is necessary for proper digestion
Multivitamin	Helps when nutritional deficiency is caused for obesity
Spirulina	High in protein, stabilizes blood sugar
Choline	Supports the body in burning fa more efficiently
BCAA	Aids in increasing growth hormone production
L-Carnitine	Break up fat deposits
L-Glutamine	Reduces sugar cravings and protect intestinal lining
Taurine	Aids in digestion of fats
DHEA	Inhibits the enzyme necessary for fat production
5-HTP	Suppresses appetite
GABA	Suppresses cravings

EFA - Essential Fatty Acids

CLA – Conjugated Linoleic Acid

BCAA – Branched Chain Amino Acids

DHEA – Dehydroepiandrosterone

5-HTP – 5-Hydroxy L-tryptophan

GABA – Gamma-Aminobutyric Acid

Herbal supplements

Herbal remedies have been utilized for centuries to cure various maladies. In the last few decades, herbal supplements were added to the market because of their efficacy in treating obesity and shrinking fat cells.

Herbs	Effects
Dandelion	Diuretic and liver protective effects – helps with weight loss
Cayenne pepper	A natural fat burner
Garcinia Cambodia	Promote fat burning and its utilization as fuel and suppresses the appetite
Green tea	High in antioxidant and aids in fat loss
Fennel	Natural appetite suppressant, aids with digestion
Turmeric	Decreases inflammation, strengthens digestion, and increases energy

Part II

Diet and Nutrition

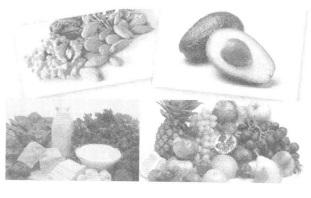

❁ ❁ ❁

Learn to eat to live and for nourishment

D iet and nutrition is the first component in your recipe for success or R4S. A well balanced diet provides the body with the nutrients it needs to stay healthy, support the immune system, and balance out hormones. Without the appropriate diet and nutrition, it is difficult to achieve all the above and attain sustainable weight loss and gain weight mastery.

Part II contains two parts, a whole foods guide and eating to nourish. You will learn the importance of whole foods in addition to acquiring the necessary knowledge on how to shop for healthy foods, prepare, cook, and eat to nourish.

Whole Foods Guide

Fruits & vegetables

Grains

Legumes & Beans

Nuts & Seeds

Dairy

Fish & Shellfish

Meat, Poultry, & Eggs

Oils/Fatty Acids

Sweeteners

Seasonings

Beverages

W hole foods are the way nature intended. They are naturally rich in the vitamins, minerals, and phytochemicals that will allow your body to function optimally and lose weight. While Part I provided the necessary knowledge about carbohydrates, proteins, and fats, Part II, breaks them down into their individual food groups to aid in making healthier choices.

Selecting wholesome food can be challenging especially because of the variety available to us. To facilitate the process, apply these simple guidelines:

- Focus on the seasons' harvest for your fruit and vegetable selections.
- Eat your grains whole and sprouted.
- Sprout your beans to reduce eructation and cooking time.
- Eat your nuts and seeds raw.
- Use dairy sparingly.
- Select wild caught fish and shellfish.
- Be lean on protein.
- Keep your oils/fatty acids essential.
- Concentrate on natural sweeteners.
- Add fresh herbs to heighten flavor and aroma.
- Drink water often.

Fruits and vegetables
"Focus on the Seasons' Harvest"

Fruits and vegetables are carbohydrates. They are most flavorful and nutritious when they are eaten in season, grown locally and organically. Spring and summer harvests are cleansing, light, juicy (due to high water content), expansive, with boundless vitamins, minerals, and phytochemicals. Autumn and winter selections are more fibrous, heavy, and compact containing less water to accommodate with the temperature. At the beginning of spring, you can indulge in fresh leaves, spring greens, sprouts, young shoots, spinach, and fresh strawberries. Summer's varieties allow for enjoyment of juicy berries, melons, corn, green beans, squashes, and many other fruits and vegetables. Autumn harvest gives us the remainder of our fruits and vegetables.

Fruits

Fruits are nature's gifts to us. Their sweetness can appease sugar cravings while providing nutrients such as antioxidant, vitamin C, and pro-vitamin A. Spring does not bring much variety as nature is reawakening from its winter slumber but what it brings are supportive to the heart and blood and can decrease symptoms of hay fever. Summer provides sweet, juicy, and bountiful fruits for all to enjoy. Autumn delivers digestive health with fibrous apples, pears, and persimmons. Winter offers immune health with citrus fruits and kiwis.

Nonetheless, you must remain mindful of how many servings of fruits you consume per day. Fruits are high in natural sugars and although better than artificial sugars, they easily increase blood sugar levels and may cause lipogenesis and oppose lipolysis when consumed heavily. Until you achieve your weight loss goal, keep your daily servings of fruits per day to a minimal and eat them preferably in the morning and early afternoon.

A few recommendations:

- ◆ Enjoy fruits at their most natural state, unprocessed and raw.
- ◆ Select unsulfured dried fruits.
- ◆ Choose seasonal and local fruits.
- ◆ Avoid canned fruits in heavy syrup.
- ◆ Avoid excessive consumption of fruit juices, which are high in sugar.

Selections

Spring	Summer	Autumn	Winter
Avocado	Berries	Apples	Oranges
Mango	Cherries	Grapes	Grapefruits
Pineapple	Peaches	Pears	Lemons
Rhubarb	Nectarines	Persimmons	Limes
Strawberry	Melons		Kiwi
	Plums		

Vegetables

Spring and summer vegetables are uplifting, light, supportive to the organs of elimination, and high in nutrients especially vitamin C, folate, iron, antioxidants, and phytochemicals. Add artichokes, dandelion, and burdock to your daily choices to aid in spring detoxification and leafy greens to aid with the summer's heat.

A few recommendations:

- ◆ Increase raw vegetable intake by adding fresh salads and other non-starchy vegetables at every meal. (Note: if you haven't consumed raw vegetables in a while, begin with one to two servings a day then slowly increase to more servings to prevent uncomfortable bloating and gas.)
- ◆ Do not overcook your vegetables. Steam or lightly sauté vegetables to decrease nutrient lost through cooking.

- Add sea vegetables. They contain minerals such as iodine and iron. Iodine increases thyroid function, which help with metabolism and weight loss. (Caution: if you've been diagnosed with hyperthyroidism avoid eating sea vegetables).

- Refrain from eating canned vegetables as they are devoid of nutrients.

Selections

Non-Starchy Vegetables	Leafy Vegetables	Herbs
Artichokes	Alfalfa sprouts	Basil
Asparagus	Arugula	Borage
Beets	Beet greens	Chives
Bell peppers	Boy choy	Cilantro
Broccoli	Broccoli raab	Dill
Carrots	Cabbage	Fennel
Cauliflower	Chard	Lemon balm
Celery	Dandelion	Mint
Eggplants	Kale	Parsley
Green garlic	Lettuce	Tarragon
Green beans	Mesclun mix	Thyme
Leeks	Mustard greens	
Onions	Spinach	
Peas	Spring greens	
Radishes	Swiss chard	
Ramps	Turnip	
Shallots	Wheat grass	

What's in season in your area?

I highly recommend eating locally and seasonally. To obtain information on what is grown in your area:

- Drive to a local farm and peek at what's growing.

- Go to your local farmer's market and speak to the grocer. He/she should have a wealth of information on seasonal harvests.

◆ Take field walks to note what's growing wild in your area (your yard is a great place to start). The plants and weeds growing wild tell a great tale on what's necessary to stay healthy. For instance, green onions and dandelion greens are the most recognizable wild greens in the grass or field in the spring. They both play important roles in supporting the liver in detoxification and decreasing allergic responses at the beginning of spring.

◆ Botanical gardens are great reference points as well. Visit your local botanical garden to gain knowledge on the plants native to your area.

Caution: Prior to picking any plants out of any yard or field, make sure the area is safe and away from high traffic and industrial pollution. DO NOT ingest plants you do not recognize. Although I do believe that uncultivated fruits and vegetables aid in maintaining health especially for the area where you reside, I however, would strongly suggest that you do your research prior to consuming any wild plants.

Grains
"Eat them whole and sprouted"

Grains are starchy carbohydrates. They are wildly distributed in the U.S. and around the world. Although grains provide natural vitamins, minerals, protein, and fiber, I do not recommend eating too much grains especially in the spring and summer months. Grains are heavy and more contracting than expanding. They increase blood viscosity and do not promote lipolysis (fat break down). However, if you would like to include grains in the diet, it is important to eat sprouted and a variety of grains to prevent wheat allergies.

Always select "**whole**" over "**refined**" grains

Whole grains vs. Refined grains

♦ Whole grains are the entire seed of the plant. They contain the germ, endosperm, and bran. They are comprised of natural vitamins, minerals, and fiber.

♦ Refined grains are milled, a process that removes the bran and germ. It is implemented to give grains a finer texture and increase shelf life, but the process strips them of nutrients such as vitamin B, iron, and dietary fiber. Synthetic vitamins and minerals are then added to compensate for the nutrients lost.

Select whole grains

Whole grains	Refined grains
Amaranth	White bread
Barley	White flour
Brown rice	White rice
Buckwheat	Pasta
Bulgur	Cereals
Couscous	Crackers
Millet	
Oats	
Quinoa	

The Process of sprouting:

1. Soak grains in water to increase moisture content and activate the phytic acid for a couple of days (rinsing and tossing out the old water daily).
2. On the last day, rinse, drain, and maintain soaked grains in a jar with a screen or mesh lid for 1-3 days. Grains will begin to form sprouts (small shoots) within 1-2 days of sprouting.
3. Sprouted grains can be eaten raw, lightly cooked, or ground into flour.

Legumes / Beans
"Better when sprouted"

Legumes are starchy carbohydrates in which the seeds are grown in pods. They are the energy storehouse of the plant. They are low in fats and cholesterol but high in carbohydrates, fiber, and protein, which make them ideal for vegetarians. When beans are not sprouted, they have similar qualities as grains. They are very contracting and heavy and tend to increase blood viscosity.

A few recommendations:

- ♦ Soak your beans overnight prior to cooking to cut down on cooking time and decrease bloating and gas formation.

- ♦ Sprout your beans (see instructions under the process of sprouting in the grains section above). Sprouting revives the nutrients in the plants, increases assimilation, changes the protein content, and decreases the amount of starch. After sprouting, you can eat your beans raw in salads, steamed, or cooked lightly.

Legumes Options

Legumes
Beans (navy, white, red, lentils, adzuki, lima)
Soybeans & soybeans products
(tofu, tempeh, soymilk & cheese, burgers)
Peas (Green peas, chickpeas, black eye peas)
Peanuts

Nuts and Seeds
"Eat them raw"

Nuts and seeds are primarily fats, although, they contain both proteins and carbohydrates as well. They are high in vitamin E, minerals, EFAs (essential fatty acids), and the amino acid arginine. Since they are more contracting in nature, they should be consumed in lower quantities and mostly as snacks.

A few recommendations:

- Eat raw nuts and seeds. They are healthier in their natural form.
- Refrain from eating salted, sugarcoated, or roasted nuts and seeds. They add extra fat and are lower in vitamins and minerals.
- Select freshly ground and non-hydrogenated nut butters. Hydrogenation alters the monounsaturated oil in nuts forming cholesterol and raising saturated fats.
- Raw nuts can also be soaked or sprouted, which tend to decrease the fat content and increase the available protein. (To sprout, simply soak nuts in water overnight. The following day, toss out water, rinse, and enjoy. You can make your own almond milk after soaking.)

Nuts and Seeds options

Nuts	Seeds
Almonds	Chia
Brazil nuts	Flax
Hazelnuts	Pumpkin
Pecans	Sesame
Walnuts	Sunflower
Cashews	

Dairy

"Eat them sparingly"

Dairy products are rich sources of protein, calcium, phosphorus, B vitamins, biotin, selenium, zinc, and potassium. They are high in fats both saturated and trans- fats as well as unsaturated fats. Fermented milk and yogurts contain health-promoting bacteria, which may help with digestion. However, dairy products are super allergenic and can cause respiratory and digestive discomforts. When consumed in excessively high quantities, they can lead to heart disease, stroke, asthma, arthritis, and obesity.

A few recommendations:

- Choose certified raw milk, cheese, and yogurt free of hormones and antibiotics.

- Choose goat dairy products, which are easier to digest and more closely resemble human protein.

- Add dairy alternatives.

- Increase other foods high in calcium such as dark leafy and non-starchy green vegetables.

- Eat dairy sparingly to maintain normal cholesterol and triglyceride levels.

Dairy options

Dairy products	Dairy alternatives	Foods high in calcium
Cheese	Almond milk & cheese	Collards
Ice cream	Soy milk & cheese	Beans
Milk	Tofu	Kale
Sour cream	Rice milk & cheese	Mustard greens
Yogurt	Brazil nut cheese	Sea vegetables
	Nutritional yeast	

Fish and Shellfish
"Select Wild Caught"

Fish and shellfish provide excellent high quality lean protein. They are high in essential fatty acids (omega 3 and omega 6 FA), vitamins B12, B6, B3, and D, and minerals like selenium, phosphorus, and potassium. They protect against cardiovascular, autoimmune, and inflammatory diseases as well as cancers. By raising HDL cholesterol levels, they shield the heart and arteries from atherosclerosis.

A few recommendations:

- Select wild caught instead of farm raised fish.
- Refrain from eating farm raised fish altogether. They tend to be lower in total EFAs and many other beneficial nutrients and are usually fed a poor diet.
- Choose smaller and deep ocean water fish instead of large and surface dwellers, which are higher in mercury content.
- Stay away from tilapia since it is a fabricated fish.
- Steam, bake, or grill your fish to retain their nutritional values.
- Shellfish tend to be higher in cholesterol content, eat them sparingly.

Your wild caught Options:

Fish	Shellfish
Alaskan salmon (pink, sockeye, or coho)	Crab
Anchovies	Lobster
Cod	Oyster
Herring	Mussels
Mackerel	Scallops
Sardines	
Snapper (Red and yellow)	
Striped bass	

Meats, Poultry, and Eggs
"Be lean on protein"

Animal flesh and eggs provide high content of readily available protein, vitamin B12, and minerals such as zinc and selenium. Since they are thermic in nature and with less accessible energy, they are a wonderful addition to the diet to facilitate weight loss. However, both animal flesh and eggs increase LDL cholesterol levels, which may lead to heart disease, stroke, and certain cancers when consumed in high quantities. Thus, it is wise to choose leaner cuts of meats, which are lower in saturated fats and cholesterol.

A few recommendations:

- ◆ Select organic and grass fed meats.
- ◆ Select lean cuts meats without fats.
- ◆ Add a variety of lean protein to your diet.
- ◆ Choose free roaming / cage free poultry. Cage-free animals experience healthier, less stressful living conditions resulting in better quality of food.
- ◆ Choose animal products not injected with antibiotics and hormones.
- ◆ Avoid animal flesh with high fat.

Your options

Red Meat	Poultry	Game
Beef	Chicken	Deer
Buffalo	Duck	Rabbit
Goat	Hen	Wild boar
Lamb	Turkey	Wild birds
Pork		

Oils / Fatty acids

"Focus on Essential Fatty Acids"

Good oils are great sources of essential fatty acids (omega 3 and omega 6 fatty acids). "Cold-pressed" oils are better than heat-pressed oils. Cold-pressed oils retain their vitamin E and antioxidants whereas heat-pressed do not. Furthermore, heat-pressed oils are treated with petroleum-derived solvents, are bleached, and deodorized.

A few recommendations:

+ Store oils in the refrigerator to prevent spoilage due to oxidation from heat and light.
+ Choose fresh, unrefined, and cold pressed oils.
+ Select oils from fish, nuts, and vegetables.
+ Limit/eliminate consumption of solid fats (lard and margarine), trans fats, hydrogenated oils, and cottonseed oils. These oils have been linked to arteriosclerosis and many other health issues.
+ Do no heat polyunsaturated oils such as flaxseed, safflower, and sunflower seed oils. Heating encourages rancidity and free radical production.
+ For cooking and baking use olive, macadamia nut oil, coconut oil, sesame oil, or canola oils.
+ For frying use canola, coconut, or grapeseed oils more heat resistant.
+ Add flax seed oil to salads, steamed vegetables, and smoothies.
+ Add a variety of "essential FA" from omega 3, 6, & 9.

Fatty acids (FA) options

Omega 3 FA	Omega 6 FA	Mono-Unsaturated FA	Saturated FA
Salmon	Safflower oil	Almond oil	Butter
Trout	Sunflower oil	Canola oil	Lard
Mackerel	Pumpkin seed oil	Olive oil	Coconut oil
Cod liver oil	Soybean oil		Cottonseed oils
Flax seed oil	Sesame seed oil		Eggs
	Walnut oil		Margarine
			Milk
			Palm kernel oil

Sweeteners

"Natural, just like Mother Nature Intended"

Sweeteners are carbohydrates and mostly simple sugars. They provide immediate energy for the brain. Unfortunately, excessive sugar intake has been a major contributor to diabetes and inflammation. Sweeteners should be utilized sparingly to avoid excess calories and fat break down opposition. You have choices when it comes to sweeteners so choose wisely.

A few recommendations:

◆ Select unrefined sugars (a list is provided below) as they are better recognizable by the body and most do not contain undesired chemicals.

◆ Avoid refined sugars such as white sugars, sugar substitutes, and artificial sugars like nutrisweet.

◆ Sweeteners add extra calories, do not over consume. Try drinking your coffee black and your tea without any sweeteners.

Sweeteners options

Unrefined	Refined (stay away from)
Agave nectar	Fructose corn syrup
Beet sugar	NutriSweet
Date sugar	Sweet'N low
Brown rice syrup	Splenda
Dried cane sugar	
Fruit juice concentrate	
Honey	
Molasses	
Pure maple syrup	
Stevia	

Seasonings
"Add variety from fresh herbs"

Seasonings add taste and flavor to food. Salt and pepper are the most commonly utilized spices; broaden your kitchen and enhance flavor by adding a variety of seasonings from fresh herbs and citrus fruits.

A few recommendations:

+ Choose sea salt instead of iodized salt.
+ Choose peppercorn medley.
+ Use cayenne pepper to replace black pepper in certain meals.
+ Select a variety of herbs to flavor your food.

Seasonings options

Common spices	Herbs	Citrus
Sea salt	Basil	Lemon & zest
Cracked peppercorn	Chili peppers	Lime & zest
Cayenne pepper	Cilantro	Orange & zest
Paprika	Dill	
Garlic	Mint	
	Oregano	
	Parsley	
	Rosemary	
	Sage	
	Thyme	

Beverages
"Make water your #1 Beverage"

Your #1 selection for beverages is pure water. However, you can add freshly extracted fruit and vegetable juices, non-caffeinated and unsweetened teas, diluted 100% juice, and infused water. No soda pop allowed.

Eating to Nourish

Shopping
Selecting
Preparing
Cooking
Combining
Timing
Eating

Food is made to nourish. It fuels the body and keeps the organs healthy and well. The "right foods" (whole foods) give your body what it needs to sustain health and growth while aiding in weight maintenance. The "wrong foods" (sugary, processed, heavy, fast and fatty foods) rob the body of essential nutrients, cause excessive weight gain, and place great burdens on the organs and the immune system. Continuous consumption of the "wrong foods" in high quantity can lead to heart disease, inflammation, cancer, obesity, hypertension, diabetes, and autoimmune illnesses.

Various factors play key roles in food assimilation and nourishment:

- Food shopping
- Food selection
- Food preparation and Cooking
- Food combining
- Timing
- Eating

Food Shopping

Shopping is the first relationship you form with your food and should not be done in a haste. Designate a set time at the beginning of the week to go shopping for the groceries you will need for that particular week. The choices you make will help you maintain your weight loss goals or steer you away from them.

How to shop:

+ Shop with a grocery list.

+ Shop locally and seasonally. Seasonal fruits and vegetables are higher in quality and nutritional content.

+ Always shop the perimeter of the grocery store first where you will find fresh fruits, vegetables, meats, and seafood. Processed foods are often located in the center aisles, stay away!

+ Use your senses to navigate around all your options.

+ Shop weekly for fresh produce (Always choose fresh first before frozen or canned).

+ Do not substitute value for price and vice versa.

+ Never go shopping on an empty stomach. Hunger navigates you towards sugary treats and processed foods.

+ Read your labels to make better selections.

Reading Labels

Reading your food labels is a part of shopping. The food label identifies information about the product including nutrition facts, ingredients, and net weight. The ingredients are listed from high to low, where the highest content is listed first and the least is listed last.

+ Take the time to read the labels.

+ Choose smaller ingredient lists, the less the better.

- Stay away from ingredients you can't pronounce or are not familiar with.
- Watch out for food additives- preservatives and dyes, artificial flavors, hydrogenated oils, and high fructose corn syrup.

Knowing how to read and interpret food labels will help you select the appropriate foods that will contribute to overall health and wellness.

Food Additives:

There are approximately 14,000 different types of additives. The "Standard American Diet" includes 3-5 pounds of these additives per year, which may not be all listed on the food label.

What are they?

They are substances added to food during manufacturing to increase the appeal of the finished product. They alter taste, texture, color, and stability of foods to prevent or reduce spoilage time. Additives can be toxic to the body and can give rise to a number of symptoms including depression, mental confusion, bi-polar disorders, headaches, abnormal nerve reflexes, and insomnia.

Preservatives:

Preservatives are added to expand shelf-life and steadiness of certain foods. They tend to accumulate in body fat causing weight gain and an array of conditions. Skin rash or hives is the most common type of allergic reactions.

Preservatives	Food Sources	Possible Effects
Acacia Gum	Chewing gum, candies, frosting, soft drinks, jellies	Asthma attacks, pregnancy fetal development problems, and skin rashes

Alginic Acid	Ice cream and other frozen desserts, salad dressing, cheese spreads and dips	Pregnancy complications and birth defects
Aspartame	Diet and sugar free soft drinks, gum, candy, instant desserts, and sweeteners	Depression, headaches, nausea, insomnia, brain damage, rashes
Benzoic Acid	Margarine, beer, pickled vegetables, soft drinks, jelly, jams, fruit juice, BBQ sauce, Fish and Shellfish	Asthma attacks, eye and mucous irritation, rashes
BHA (Butylated hydroxyanisole) **BHT** (Butylated hydroxytoluene)	Chewing gum, candy breakfast cereal, sausage, desserts; oil containing products: potato chips, vegetable oils, and shortening	High cholesterol, infertility, organ damage, immune disorders, behavior problems
Irradiation (Picowaved)	spices, chicken, fruits and vegetables	Cancer
Monosodium Glutamate (MSG)	Chinese food, condiments, salt substitutes, soups, seasonings	Allergies, chest tightness, diarrhea, headaches, eye inflammation
Nitrites / Nitrates	Processed meats, bacon, ham, sausages, smoked meats, cold cuts meats, hot dogs	Stomach Cancer, birth defects, childhood leukemia
Saccharin	Sugar free sweeteners, soft drinks	Cancer
Salicylates	Spices: curry powder, paprika, thyme, dill, oregano, and turmeric; Prepared foods: Cake mixes, pudding, ice cream, gum, soft drinks and most dried fruits and berries.	Allergic reactions
Sulfur Dioxide, Bisulfite & Sulfites	Dried fruits, shrimp, frozen potatoes, wine	Allergies and asthma attacks
Tertiary Butydroquinone (TBHG)	Baking sprays, candy bars, fast foods	Behavioral problems

Dyes:

Artificial dyes are extensively utilized in foods, beverages, drugs, and cosmetics to enhance their colors. Most artificial dyes are petroleum products derived from coal tar. There are many known coloring agents. The following are the most commonly used.

Dyes	Food Sources	Possible Effects
Blue No. 2	Cat food and soda pop	Brain cancer
Citrus red	Florida oranges	Cancer
Green No. 3	Lime drinks and popsicles	Thyroid cancer
Yellow No. 5	Orange drinks: Tang, Daybreak, Awake; Royal and Jell-O gelatin desserts; Kraft Italian dressing and Mac & cheese; Pillsbury, Duncan Hines Cake mixes and icing; French's seasoning salt	Allergic responses and attention deficit disorder (ADHD)
Yellow No. 6	Soda pop and candy	kidney cancer, adrenal damage, allergies
Red No. 40	Bake goods, candy, cereal	Allergic responses, cancer, hyperactivity in children

High fructose corn syrup:

High fructose corn syrup (HFCS) is a sweetener made from corn. It comes in two compositions – HFCS 42 and HFCS 55 meaning. HFCS 42 is composed of 42% fructose and 58% glucose whereas HFCS 55 contains 55% fructose and 45% glucose. They are both utilized as primary or secondary ingredients in processed foods such as breads, salad dressings, condiments, cakes, cookies, crackers, and many other unsuspected products. For health and weight loss, avoid foods with HFCS as their primary ingredient.

Food Selection

Food selection can be an intimidating process because of the variety available to you. Now that you have better knowledge of food shopping, selecting proper foods may become easier. Remember to always navigate towards the perimeter of the store first before making any selections.

Select:

- Whole foods that are free of artificial flavors, colors, and high fructose corn syrup.
- Vegetables and fruits that look and feel fresh with vibrant and inviting colors.
- Meats that do not look old or spoil, or smell rotten.
- Organic, cage free, and minimally processed meats and poultry whenever possible. They are not only free of chemicals, pesticides, herbicides, and fungicides but they tend to be more flavorful and higher in nutrients compared to conventionally grown foods.
- Wild caught seafood over farm-raised.
- Raw and shelled nuts.
- Highly nutritious foods that will cleanse the blood, allow the body to release toxins, and shrink fat cells.

Food Preparation

Preparing and cooking your selected food items are other experiences of the senses. Using your eyes, nose, ears, and mouth will activate the salivary glands and prepare your stomach for digestion. You should schedule time for food preparation at the beginning of the week to assure success and to prevent starvation and overeating.

Here are a few tips:

- All vinaigrette can be prepared ahead of time and stored in the refrigerator.

- Prepare and cook most of your protein at the beginning of each week by following the recipes outlined in the recipe section.

- Separate your cooked proteins into 3-6 ounces and store in the refrigerator.

- Grab a large glass bowl with a lid and prepare a week's worth of salad. (To prevent your leafy green vegetables from turning brown too quickly, tear them with your fingers instead of cutting them with a knife. The blade causes oxidation to occur more rapidly.)

- Bag your vegetables for stir frying, steaming, or grilling so you can just grab and cook.

- Bag your morning smoothie ingredients for convenience.

- Whenever possible, weigh all proteins cooked and all vegetables raw.

Cooking

While cooking, keep in mind that your emotions can transfer into the food and affect taste and digestibility. Don't cook while you're angry, frustrated, and generally unhappy. Cook with love and pleasure. In addition, cook in a way that preserves most of the vitamins and minerals in the foods.

- Eat vegetables raw (mostly), lightly steamed, sautéed, or roasted. *Note: as soon as a vegetable is harvested it begins to lose nutrients (vitamins and minerals). Eat vegetables within a week of purchase.*

- Bake, grill, steam, or sear animal protein.

- Sprout, then steam whole grains such as rice and quinoa (use a rice cooker if possible).

- Sprout beans before cooking to reduce cooking time but increase assimilation.

Food combining

It is very important to know how to combine your food for better digestion, optimal health, and sustainable weight loss. Some foods such as melons digest very rapidly and when combined with other foods they slow down their digestion and cause fermentation. Fats digest slowly and cause an arrest in other food digestion.

In addition, different foods require different stomach pH for digestion. For instance, protein requires a more acidic pH for metabolism whereas carbohydrates require a more alkaline pH. Thus, eating them in the right order will improve digestion. Your order of eating should be:

- **First**: Proteins (meat, fish, shellfish)
- **Second**: Fats (oils, nuts)
- **Third**: Starches (potatoes, bread, grains)
- **Fourth**: Salads (leafy greens, non-starchy vegetables)
- **Fifth**: Fruits (bananas, berries, citrus fruits)
- **Last**: Desserts (pies, cakes, ice cream)

Eating your protein first allow the acidic medium that the protein requires for digestion to be secreted. Since carbohydrates are digested in a more alkaline pH, they can disrupt protein digestion and should be eaten after proteins and fats.

Proper food combining:	Poor food combining:
Enhances digestion Helps the body function better Increases energy level Promotes health and vitality	Decreases nutrient absorption and assimilation Causes intestinal bloating, gas, and dysbiosis Increases abdominal discomforts and fat

Which foods combine well and which foods do not?

Food Group	☑ Combine ☒ Do not combine
Proteins All meats, poultry, fish, eggs, soy products, legumes	☑ Leafy greens and Non-starchy vegetables (one protein per meal, two max) ☒ Starches such as steak and potatoes ☒ Two or more proteins at once (e.g. steak and shrimp) - harder on the digestive system
High fat proteins Nuts, seeds, dairy products	☑ Acid-fruits, leafy greens, non-starchy vegetables ☒ Sweet fruits and starches
Fats and oils Avocado, cream, butter, sour cream, and oils (flax, olive, sesame, etc.)	☑ Acid-fruits, leafy greens, non-starchy vegetables, starches Eat in smaller quantities ☒ Proteins (e.g., fries & hamburgers – fats inhibit gastric juices which slows down protein digestion)
Starches Potato, sweet potato, beet, carrot, pumpkin, parsnip, bread, pasta, rice	☑ All other vegetables and Fats ☒ Proteins
Leafy greens Bok choy, chard, cabbage, parsley, spinach, lettuce, kale ...	☑ All foods
Non-starchy vegetables Celery, cucumber, broccoli, cauliflower, onions, radish, ...	☑ All foods
Sweet fruits Banana, dates, figs, persimmon, all dried foods	☑ Sub-acid fruits, lettuce and celery ☒ Acid fruits, proteins, and starches
Sub-acid fruits Apple, apricot, berries, cherry, grape, nectarine peach, papaya, pear, plum, mango	☑ Sweet and acid fruits, lettuce and celery
Acid fruits Lemon, lime, orange, grapefruit, pineapple, tomato, strawberry, kiwi, pomegranate	☑ Sub-acid fruits, fats, oils, and nuts. ☒ Never with sweet fruits, ☒ Animal proteins

| Melons | ☑ Only with other melons |
| Cantaloupe, honeydew, watermelon | ☒ Other fruits, meats, fats, etc. |

Mealtime

Eating at the appropriate time is a great approach to increased metabolism and successful weight loss. Unless you are fasting, do not take too long in between meals to eat or wait until your body exhibits severe signs of hunger such as headache, weariness, dizziness, irritability, diminished concentration, fatigue, and/or clumsiness to grab a bite to eat. In fact, you should schedule in mealtime daily to accelerate your metabolism and eating every 2-3 hours may facilitate the process.

Furthermore, timing is of utmost importance after exercise. Eat within 30 minutes to 1 hour after exercising to allow muscle repair and rebuilding of new muscle fibers to occur. You can drink a post-workout protein shake immediately, or eat a prepared meal with adequate amount of protein.

Eating

Before Eating

Before you eat:

- Drink 10 ounces of water at least 10 minutes before you eat to satiate any thirst and clean your palate.
- Arrange your plate so it can look appealing to the eyes, which may stimulate the salivary glands to produce more saliva and increase digestion.
- Find a place to seat comfortably to prepare your body for digestion.
- Prior to your first bite, relax yourself and allow clear and happy thoughts to infiltrate your mind.

Eating:

Since food is made to nourish, the food you ingest should feed and nourish every cell in your body, so it is very important to eat in a way that stimulates digestion and allow food to be distributed properly.

A few recommendations:

- **Chew, chew, and chew as much as possible**. Digestion starts in the mouth. Hence, chewing reduces the break down time in the stomach, decreases the workload on the body, and begins extracting nutrients out of the food prior to reaching your stomach and intestines. You should chew a minimum of 22 times before swallowing.

- **Take smaller bites**. Smaller bites allow saliva, which is filled with enzymes, to mix well with the food in your mouth and commence the break down process.

- **Do not engage in unpleasant arguments or discussions**. This may cause digestive disturbances. You should feel happy and be ready to delight in your food.

- **Enjoy** your food thoroughly.

- **Do not refill your plate** until you have sat for at least 10-15 minutes to facilitate communication between your brain and stomach. It takes a few minutes for your stomach to signal your brain that you're full.

After eating:

What you do after you eat is as important as the other two, before eating and eating. Final digestion occurs after eating. Therefore,

- Relax for a few minutes to facilitate better digestion.
- Clear the table and happily wash the dishes ☺.
- Engross in pleasant conversations, watch a movie, or take a walk outside.

- Do not engage in heavy exercises immediately after eating. Exercise takes blood away from the digestive track to distribute it to the muscles and the heart, which disrupts digestion.
- Do not lay down or go to sleep. When you lay down, stomach acid can rush back into the esophagus causing heartburn.
- Drink 10 ounces of water, 10 minutes after eating to fill your belly and avoid overeating and/or second helpings.

Part III

Physical Activity

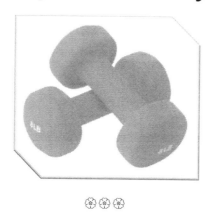

✿ ✿ ✿

Physical activity has been known to cause uncontrollable happiness and optimal health.

E xercise is the second most important component in R4S since it is, undeniably, indispensable to weight loss and overall health. Starting an exercise regimen is easy maintaining it is more difficult because it takes:

- Discipline
- Perseverance
- Dedication
- Determination
- Strong will
- A vision and a plan

To succeed, you must make a commitment to yourself, follow through on all promises, and perform exercises you enjoy.

Types of Exercises

Cardiovascular
Strength Training
Interval Training
Flexibility

A healthy and successful weight loss program always incorporates exercise because of all the benefits it provides. For example, exercise:

- Accelerates metabolism and lean body mass.
- Reduces body fat, cholesterol, and blood pressure.
- Improves glucose and insulin metabolism.

- Enhances mood, energy, and quality of sleep.
- Decreases stress.
- Improves lymph and blood circulation
- Increases detoxification of stored toxins.

However, the benefits of exercise only last as long as you continue to make exercise a priority and a daily part of your healthy lifestyle. Select activities you enjoy and are willing to commit to long-term. Having an accountability partner, a reliable workout associate, a personal trainer, or a fitness group may be just what you need to maintain a regular exercise routine and follow through on your promises.

Caution: Prior to starting any exercise program, consult with your healthcare provider.

You should adhere to three major components when beginning any exercise program:

1) Frequency,
2) Intensity, and
3) Time

This applies to both aerobic (running, swimming) and anaerobic (strength training). You can vary any of these components one at a time when you desire to increase endurance or get over a plateau. For instance, if you have been following a regular routine for 3-4 weeks and you are no longer seeing results, you can increase your workout frequency to surpass your plateau while keeping your intensity and time the same. This will prevent exhaustion and/or injury. You can begin to change the intensity or duration of your workout once you have stabilized the frequency for at least two weeks.

When you are starting an exercise regimen, keep in mind that you do have options. You can concentrate on cardiovascular solely or combine cardiovascular, calisthenics, and weight training for best results. Flexibility training should always be a part of your routine and every workout should include a warm-up and a cool down.

Warm Up and Cool Down

Before and after you exercise, it is important to properly warm-up and cool-down your muscles and joints to prevent harm and the excessive soreness that follows a good workout.

Warm-up

Your warm up should last 5-10 minutes, mimic the activity that you are about to perform, and engage larger muscle groups like the hamstrings and quadriceps but at a much lower intensity. Walking, gentle gliding on the elliptical, and riding a bicycle on low speed are all examples of warm-up exercises. Warm up increases circulation throughout the body and prepares it for a more intense and better workout. Stretch for another 5 to 10 minutes as part of your warm-up and never stretch a cold muscle.

Cool-Down

A well-performed cool down immediately following your workout, reduces muscle tightness and soreness, redistributes blood flow to other areas, and lengthens muscle fibers. A cool-down should last 5-10 minutes follow by at least 5 minutes of stretching.

Cardiovascular Training

Cardiovascular (cardio) exercise is any exercise that increases your heart rate. It utilizes larger muscle movement over a sustained period of time. You should aim for a minimum of 30 minutes of cardio per day and reach 55 to 85 percent of your maximum heart rate (MHR) for best results.

What is MHR?

MHR is the upper limit of what your cardiovascular system can handle during strenuous physical activity. To calculate your MHR simply subtract your age from 220.

MHR = 220-age

If you are 40 years of age, your maximum heart rate is 180. Your recommended target range is between 99 and 153 beats per minute.

Examples of cardiovascular exercises:

Cardio Exercises
Jogging
Running
Bicycling
Swimming
Stair climbing
Dancing
Hiking
Playing sports

Strength Training

Strength training refers to any exercise that uses some form of resistance to strengthen and build muscle. During strength training exercises, you can use free weights and /or machines (weight training), resistance bands, resistance balls, and/or your own body weight (calisthenics, yoga, Pilates).

1. Weight Training

Weight training is a type of strength training that utilizes weights for resistance. Weight training increases muscle tone and improves overall appearance. Weight training can be performed with free weights (barbells and dumbbells) and/or machines.

Some tips for beginners:

♦ Start with one exercise per muscle group then steadily increase (e.g., bench press for upper body and squats for lower body).

♦ Once you move to two exercises per muscle group, train agonist muscles together and antagonist muscles together (e.g., work **biceps and back** on the same day and **triceps & chest** on the same day).

♦ Always start with a weight you can do 8-12 repetitions with (e.g., 20lbs), but are fatiguing by the 12th rep. If the 12th rep does not fatigue your muscle, increase to a higher weight.

♦ Do not train on cold muscles. Always start with a 5 min warm-up and end with a 5 min cool down.

If you combine cardio with weight training, always perform your weight training first before your cardio to facilitate a better workout, decrease muscle fatigue, burn more calories, and attain the most from your workout.

Follow these guidelines:

Time	Exercise
5 min	Warm-up
20-30 min	Weight training
30-45 min	Cardio
5 min	Cool down

Examples of basic weight training exercises:

	Exercises	Main muscle worked	Other muscle worked
Back	Lat pull down Seated row Back extensions	Latissimus dorsi	Biceps Middle back
Biceps	Bicep curls Hammer curls	Biceps	Brachioradialis
Chest	Chest/bench press Push ups Flys	Chest	Triceps Shoulders & Pec muscles
Shoulders	Military press Lateral & front raise	Shoulders	Triceps
Triceps	Triceps dips Triceps pushdown Overhead extension	Triceps	Chest Shoulders
Legs	Squats Lunges	Quadriceps	Hamstring Calves Glutes
Abs	Crunches Sit-ups Leg lifts	Abdominal muscles	Lower back

2. Calisthenics

Calisthenics aka body-weight training, are exercises consisting of gross motor movements performed to develop strength and flexibility using one's own body instead of specialized equipment.

Calisthenics Exercises

Upper body	Core	Lower body
Pushups Pull-ups Dips	Crunches Sit-ups Leg raises Plank	Squats Jump squats Lunges Jumping jacks Calf-raises

3. Yoga and Pilates (see definition in the flexibility section)

Interval training

Interval training is characterized by short bursts of vigorous physical activity intermixed with periods of rest or low-intensity.

What are some benefits of interval training over regular cardio?

Interval training:

- Improves aerobic and anaerobic capacity
- Reduces abdominal fat
- Burns more calories
- Increases metabolism
- Prevents boredom
- Inhibits plateau
- Transforms physique more rapidly

Interval training can carry a higher risk for injury, especially if you are at the beginner level. Always start slow and at your fitness level while challenging your body. It is very rewarding. Do not give up and you will reap the benefits. Drink plenty of water before during and after your training.

Cardio Interval training

Track, trail, or Treadmill Interval training

Beginner

Time (min)	Activity	Speed on Treadmill
0:00-5:00	Warm-up, easy- moderate pace	3.0-3.5 mph
5:00-6:00	Light Jog	4.0 mph
6:00-7:00	Jog	4.5 mph
7:00-8:00	Fast Jog	5.0 mph
8:00-9:00	Run	5.5 mph
9:00-10:00	Active rest (walk)	2.0 mph
10:00-15:00	Repeat from 5:00-10:00 min	4.0-6.0 mph
15:00-20:00	Cool Down	3.5-3.0 mph

Advanced

Time (min)	Activity	Speed on Treadmill
0:00-5:00	Warm-up, Moderate to fast pace walk	3.5-4.0 mph
5:00-6:00	Fast Jog	5.5 mph
6:00-7:00	Run	6.0 mph
7:00-8:00	Run	6.5 mph
8:00-9:00	Sprint	7.0 mph
9:00-10:00	Active rest (walk)	3.0 mph
10:00-15:00	Repeat from 5:00-10:00 min	4.0-7.0 mph
15:00-20:00	Cool Down	3.5-4.0 mph

*If the speed is too fast at the beginning, you can scale down to a more comfortable speed and increase as you improve.

Calisthenics / Cardio / Abs - High Intensity Interval Training (HIIT)

Your options include 15 seconds, 20 seconds, 30 seconds, and 1 minute each of HIIT. Each variety targets and strengthens different muscle groups. For instance, HIIT 1 is all about increasing endurance and strengthening the lungs and the heart, HIIT 2 strengthens the leg muscles, HIIT 3 targets arms and chest, and HIIT 4 supports the core muscles (abs and lower back).

15 seconds each HIIT

1 minute rest after each round

Time	HIIT 1	HIIT 2	HIIT 3	HIIT 4
5 min	Warm-up	Warm-up	Warm-up	Warm-up
15 sec	Jump rope	Front kicks	Triceps dips	Crunches
15 sec	Jump. Jacks	Squats	Burpees	Sit-ups
15 sec	High knees	Side kicks	Climbers	Leg lifts
15 sec	Butt kicks	Alt. Lunges	Pushups	Plank
1 min	Rest	Rest	Rest	Rest
5 min	Cool-down	Cool-down	Cool-down	Cool-down

Level I – 10 rounds; Level II – 15 rounds; Level III – 20 rounds

20 seconds each HIIT

1 minute rest after each round

Time	HIIT 1	HIIT 2	HIIT 3	HIIT 4
5 min	Warm-up	Warm-up	Warm-up	Warm-up
20 sec	Jump rope	Jump squats	Burpees	Crunches
20 sec	Jump. Jacks	Suicides	Pushups	Sit-ups
20 sec	High knees	Alt. Lunges	Triceps dips	Sitting twists
1 min	Rest	Rest	Rest	Rest
5 min	Cool-down	Cool-down	Cool-down	Cool-down

Level I – 10 rounds; Level II – 15 rounds; Level III – 20 rounds

30 seconds each HIIT

1 minute rest after each round

Time	HIIT 1	HIIT 2	HIIT 3	HIIT 4
5 min	Warm-up	Warm-up	Warm-up	Warm-up
30 sec	Jump rope	Jump squats	Triceps dips	Crunches
30 sec	Suicides	Alt. Lunges	Pushups	Plank
1 min	Rest	Rest	Rest	Rest
5 min	Cool-down	Cool-down	Cool-down	Cool-down

Level I – 10 rounds; Level II – 15 rounds; Level III – 20 rounds

1 minute each HIIT - 30 seconds rest between each exercise

Time	HIIT 1	HIIT 2	HIIT 3	HIIT 4
5 min	Warm-up	Warm-up	Warm-up	Warm-up
1 min	Jump rope	Suicides	Pushups	Crunches
30 sec	Rest	Rest	Rest	Rest
1 min	Jump. Jacks	Squats	Burpees	Sit-ups
30 sec	Rest	Rest	Rest	Rest
1 min	High knees	Front kicks	Climbers	Sitting twist
30 sec	Rest	Rest	Rest	Rest
1 min	Butt kicks	Alt. Lunges	Triceps dips	Leg lifts
30 sec	Rest	Rest	Rest	Rest
1 min	Sprint in place	Side kicks	Plank jacks	Side crunch
30 sec	Rest	Rest	Rest	Rest
5 min	Cool-down	Cool-down	Cool-down	Cool-down

Level I – 5 rounds; Level II – 10 rounds; Level III – 15 rounds

Find the best fit for you. You can vary your performance with cardio only, calisthenics only, abs only, cardio plus calisthenics, or a combination of all four. Start at your fitness level and level up. Continue to challenge your body and make the most out of your workout.

Your rest period is very important. You should incorporate active rest to lower your heart rate more efficiently (e.g., pacing or walking) Instead of stopping abruptly. Find a partner to work with you. A little competition can boost your self-confidence and increase fitness level.

Flexibility Training

As you begin your exercise program, it is imperative to incorporate activities that increase flexibility. You should dedicate 3-4 days out of the week for flexibility training. You can include flexibility in your warm-up and cool-down or as separate workouts.

Flexibility training can help:

♦ Prevent injury,
♦ Increase range of motion,
♦ Promote relaxation,
♦ Improve performance and posture,
♦ Reduce stress,
♦ Lengthen muscle fibers, and
♦ Keep your body feeling loose and agile

Types of flexibility training:

1. **Pilates**: a system of exercises designed to improve strength, flexibility, posture, and enhance mental awareness

2. **Static stretching**: involves a slow, gradual, and controlled elongation of the muscle through the full range of motion. The stretch is held in a challenging but comfortable position for 10-30 seconds.
3. **Qi Gong**: integrates physical postures or balance, breathing techniques, and focused intention
4. **Yoga**: incorporates controlled breathing, stretching, and simple meditation for health and relaxation

Part IV

Mind-Body Connection

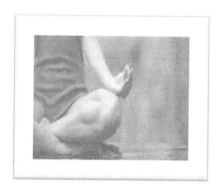

✿ ✿ ✿

"The body achieves what the mind believes." Bob Greene

M

ind-Body Connection is the third component of R4S that is often neglected or omitted in the weight loss process.

What's the link between weight loss and the mind-body connection?

Everything starts in the mind and to win at losing, the mind has to be right. You must reconnect with your whole self to allow progress to occur. Frequently, the way you see yourself, your attitude towards food and eating, and the stories you tell are great contributors to weight gain. Once you begin to form a positive relationship with the beautiful being that you are and the food you eat, weight may no longer be an issue.

In this section, you will learn to gain mastery of your mind by fostering a positive mental attitude in turn your body will collaborate with your new way of thinking and eating and yield success.

Fostering a Positive Mental Attitude

Meditation
Affirmation
Visualization
Breathing
Journaling and Self-Work
Self-Pampering
Rest and Sleep
Play and Fun

Fostering a positive mental attitude is a necessary step in the mind-body connection. As your perspectives shift, everything in your surrounding follows to support your new way of thinking and perceiving.

What are your attitude and thoughts towards food and eating?

1. Are you enjoying the food you eat?

When children are eating, they make all types of sounds or noises and/or perform their own little rhythmic dances affirming enjoyment of their foods. This simple process stimulates digestion and neurotransmitters in the brain begin to associate eating with pleasure.

What happened to that child?

As we age, most of us begin to lose that pleasant association and start linking eating and food with weight gain. The way you feel and think about food and the food you ingest play major roles in how that food will ultimately affect your body.

Have you often pondered why some naturally skinny people can eat whatever they want and not gain weight? The explanation is simple. They do not associate eating with weight gain; they eat for the pure enjoyment of eating.

Whether you are eating a salad or fries, your attitude and thoughts towards that food should be that of pure pleasure delight, and nourishment. If you carry negative emotions towards specific foods and you continue to consume them, they will affect the way your body processes and assimilates them sometimes causing indigestion, heartburn, upset stomach, and weight gain. If you make a conscious decision to eat something unhealthy, learn to love and enjoy it or do not eat it at all. However, when you begin to make better food choices your body will ask for more nourishing and uplifting foods and less processed and fast foods.

2. Are you keeping a positive mental attitude while you are eating?

Eating can be a time to reconnect with family and friends and to explore your senses, especially taste and sight. It is not the time to get into arguments, be negative about life, fussing at your children, rushing, or driving. When you sit peacefully with a positive mental attitude, your body responds better, digestion improves, and weight loss occurs. Learn to schedule "meal time" to enjoy your food fully without the desire for gorging, overeating, or shoving food in your mouth uncontrollably.

3. What are your triggers? What cause you to binge or overeat?

Take a mini assessment of your mental state before, during, and after meals to decipher your triggers and causes for binging or overeating.

Mini assessment:
- Are you eating to fill a void? Yes / No
- Are you eating because you feel depress, bothered, anxious, or lonely? Yes / No
- Are you eating because you are hungry, thirsty, or bored? Yes / No
- Are you eating to soothe or bury your emotional pain and imbalances? Yes / No
- Are you eating to feel better about yourself and circumstances? Yes / No
- Are you eating because you simply love and enjoy to eat? Yes / No

Getting to the root cause of the problem by analyzing your attitude, habits, and thoughts towards food and eating as well as figuring out your triggers can help you formulate a concrete plan of action.

I have added some methods to facilitate that process:

- Meditation
- Positive affirmations
- Visualization
- Journaling
- Seeking counsel

Whatever you do, will be a forward step towards loving your body, losing weight, and increasing overall health and wellness.

Meditation

Meditation is the process of quieting one's thoughts to allow peace, serenity, and alignment to flow. You can think of meditation as an exercise for the brain and an excellent tool to connect the body with the mind and spirit.

You should schedule in at least 10-30 minutes per day to meditate. It is best to meditate first thing in the morning since your mind is clear and your thoughts rested but anytime during the day or before bed will be beneficial.

Meditation has been proven to:

- Reduce anxiety and stress. This may help your body switch from "fight or flight" mode to a more relaxed state where digestion and assimilation can occur.
- Increase immune health to fight off illnesses and keep you healthy.

- Yield greater emotional balance to prevent overeating or hoarding.
- Allow better awareness of self and the environment to begin to connect on a much deeper level with self, others, and nature.
- Increase peace, happiness, joy, and bliss to create stability, a positive state of mind, and decrease cortisol production and inflammation.
- Generate a rise in focus and attention to set goals and achieve them.
- Improve sleep; support overall mood and weight loss.

How to meditate:

There are no set ways or rules on how to meditate, but the methods outlined below may be advantageous.

- Find a comfortable place to sit quietly without interruptions for 15-20minutes each day.
- Close your eyes and begin to quiet your mind.
- You can listen to music, sounds in the room, or repeat a mantra.
- Do not engage or participate in your thoughts; let them flow easily into the abyss.
- Keep your eyes close and sit restfully until the end of your meditation.

You are now ready to tackle your day!!!

(Follow the 21-day Meditation challenge in Phase I – Mind/Body connection section)

Affirmation

Repeating positive affirmations about yourself to yourself daily is a proven method to build self-love and self-confidence. You can begin by making statements such as,

> I love myself
>
> I love my body
>
> I am beautiful
>
> I am healthy
>
> I am perfect
>
> I am skinny
>
> I am fit
>
> I accept myself
>
> I am energetic
>
> I make healthy choices
>
> I am happy
>
> I am comfortable in my skin
>
> I love every single cell of my body

Recommendations:

- Begin your day by repeating positive affirmative words to yourself – you can either sit on your bed upon rising or in front of a mirror.

- Write the way you see yourself in your journal and change any negative views to positive ones.

- Expand on describing words that you associate with your persona.

- Repeat affirmations daily for at least 21 days – this process will help build new neuronal networks in your brain to help you believe and begin seeing yourself exactly the way you desire.

Visualization

Visualization is a powerful process that allows you to see your goals before they happen. For instance, if your goal is to be 125 lbs and you want to fit into your favorite swimsuit, begin to visualize yourself exactly how you would like to look. Imagine yourself at the beach on a beautiful sunny summer day wearing your swimsuit. You are embracing your curves and your figure looks astonishing. Create the image in your mind, feel the sensation you receive, and hold on to it. See it, be it, and feel it.

Visualization can get you to your goals faster. As you feed your brain constant images of that perfect body, ultimately it will comply.

Recommendations:

- Visualize the size you would like to be throughout the day.
- Add emotions with your visualization such as elation, excitement, happiness, etc.
- Create a vision board by cutting words and pictures out of magazines and pasting them on a poster board. If you have a younger picture of yourself at your perfect weight, cut that picture out and place it on the board along with words like beautiful, healthy, skinny, strong, perfect size, 125lbs, etc. Look at the picture daily and begin to embody that image.

(*Follow the 21-day Affirmation/Visualization challenge in Phase II – Mind/Body connection Section*)

Breathing

Breath is essential to life and essential to weight loss. When you breathe in, you inhale oxygen and when you breathe out, you exhale carbon dioxide. Therefore, breathing allows your lungs to remove toxins out of the body and bring more oxygen to the organs. The more toxins you exhale the more you shrink fat cells.

As you inhale, feel your abdomen and chest expanding to fill your lungs with air, as you exhale feel the abdomen contracting to release carbon dioxide from the lungs. That contraction strengthens core muscles and helps you build tighter abs.

Recommendations:

- Upon rising, take in slow deep breaths, inhaling through the nose and exhaling slowly out the mouth to welcome life and abundant health.

- Take moments away from noise to practice deep breathing throughout your day and allow positivity to infiltrate your being.

- Breath can facilitate a deeper self-connection and self-awareness. As you inhale, imagine breathing in health, admiration, self-confidence, love, and positivity; as you exhale, push out negativity, self-hatred, uncertainty, and doubt. Do that a few times a day.

Journaling and self-work

Frequently issues of body image, insecurities, shame, guilt, helplessness and hopelessness, lost, hate, depression, anxiety, vulnerability, and many other feelings and fears are hidden behind eating disorders, weight gain, and inability to lose weight. People often choose food to cope, soothe aches, alleviate stresses, and feel good.

Journaling is a method of self-exploration and awareness, where you invite your pen and paper to participate in free flow of ideas, thoughts, self-work, plans, goals, etc.

Recommendations:

- Purchase a journal and begin to explore your thoughts and feelings on a more intimate level.

- Write positive affirmative words in your journal daily.
- Maintain a journal of your food intake and the emotions that emerge while eating.
- Jot down your triggers- situations, people, or places- that may contribute to binge eating, constant snacking, or inability to control excessive food ingestion.
- Join a support group or seek counsel from a health care practitioner, a pastor, a friend, or family member. By resolving body image issues, you can accelerate your weight loss. ***Keep in mind you are not alone!***

(Follow the 21-day Journaling challenge in Phase I – Mind/Body connection Section)

Self-Pampering

Part of accepting and appreciating yourself is scheduling time to pamper and take care of yourself and your needs in a more loving way. No one can love you more than you can love yourself.

Recommendations:

- Schedule time to center yourself daily by meditating first thing in the morning.
- Spend time outside in nature and let the energy of the season soothe you.
- Take relaxing baths.
- Get massages often.
- Go on spiritual retreats.
- Spend time with nurturing and inspiring family members and friends.
- Remain optimistic and enjoy your life to the fullest!

(Follow the 21-day Pamper Yourself challenge in Phase III – Mind/Body connection section)

Be easy on yourself and your progress!

Keep in mind that "*Rome was not built in one day*" and it may take time to reach your final goals. If you are not seeing the progress you desire, don't give up, keep at it, and your efforts will prove beneficial overtime.

Recommendations:

- You can schedule in one day a week (perhaps Sunday or Friday) to have a small piece of your favorite dessert, a snack food, or a glass of wine to pacify your cravings. Do not overindulge, if you do, do not beat yourself up about it. Sit comfortably, relax, enjoy it, and pick up where you left off the following day.
- Take it one day at a time and do not get discouraged.
- *Remember if you fall off the wagon, you can always get back on. Tomorrow is a new day.*
- Trust in your abilities to stay true to the program and achieve your goals.

Rest & Sleep

Sleep rejuvenates and refreshes the body. The organs benefit greatly and you are aware of the difference. Did you know that sleep is valuable to weight loss? You must sleep to allow your organs to rejuvenate and lose weight.

What are some of the benefits of restful sleep?

- ✓ Improves mood; you become less irritable.
- ✓ Increases happiness and decreases depression.

- ✓ Reduces cravings especially sugar cravings.
- ✓ Decreases late night snacking.
- ✓ Upsurges focus and concentration.
- ✓ Supports digestion and equilibrium.
- ✓ Increases weight loss.

Recommendations:

- ♦ Sleep a minimum of 8 hours per night to allow your body to relax.
- ♦ Rest when you are tired.
- ♦ Take catnaps during the day.
- ♦ Plan your day accordingly and schedule in bedtime.

Fun and Play

There are endless possibilities for enjoyment and play. Fun and play are foods for the soul. When you're happy and having fun your cortisol levels (stress hormones) decrease and your endorphins (feel good hormone) increase. Your mind relaxes and your spirit is at peace.

Recommendations:

- ♦ Schedule time in your day for play and fun with family and friends.
- ♦ Visit a botanical garden, run a race, or take up a hobby.
- ♦ Go on a mountain hike.
- ♦ Make a bucket list and a plan to achieve it.
- ♦ Have fun and be happy because happiness produces favorable results.

The methods listed above will aid in developing a positive mental attitude, forming a deeper self-connection, and maintaining healthy balance and homeostasis. Choose a few of those methods and commit to them for at least 21 days. Participate in the mind-body challenges at the end of the each phase. They will prove to be extremely advantageous and facilitate self-love and acceptance.

Program overview

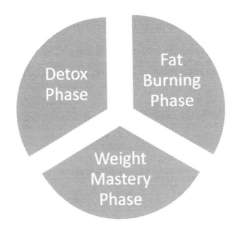

⚘ ⚘ ⚘

The key to your success is contingent on your commitment and dedication to the program.

I n the next 9 weeks, I will serve as your personal coach to help you succeed on your weight loss journey by utilizing the three components of R4S, healthy eating (HE), exercise (E), and mind-body connection (MBC). This will require **dedication, commitment, and determination**. You will get what you put in so give it your all. In the end, you will be that much closer to achieving your weight loss goals and attaining weight mastery. *You can do it, let's get started!*

Your program is divided into 3 phases, each phase lasting 21 days. Experts states, it takes 21 days to change a habit; here's your chance! Keep in mind that you can alternate between phases or prolong any favorable phase until you reach your goals.

1. **Phase I - Detox Phase**
2. **Phase II - Fat Burning Phase**
3. **Phase III – Weight Mastery / Healthy 4 Life Phase**

Diet and Nutrition Overview

1. **Detox Phase** - Remove the junk to jumpstart your weight loss.
   - In week 1, you begin by eliminating refined sugar, heavy, hyper-allergenic, fatty, and processed foods out of the diet to prepare your body for cleansing week.
   - In Week 2, you start a 7-day cleanse to rid the body of fats, toxins, and mucus, detoxify your organs so they can function optimally, jumpstart your weight loss, and set the stage for a successful weight loss program.

- In week 3, you reintroduce some of the foods eliminated during the first week to assess food allergies and prepare for fat burning phase.

2. **Fat Burning Phase** - Revive your organs to maximize fat loss

   The second phase of the program is all about maximizing on fat loss.

   - You will rid your body of the undesired fat by increasing your metabolism, reducing your net carb intake, and increasing your protein and healthy fat. This is the phase to give it your best and visualize that perfect weight at the end of these 3 weeks.
   - You can prolong this phase until you reach your weight loss goals.

3. **Weight Mastery / Healthy 4 Life Phase** - Setting the stage for sustainable weight loss.

   The last phase of the program is as important as the other 2 phases if not more. In this phase,

   - You will eat in a way to continue losing weight until you attain your desired goal weight.
   - You will incorporate what you've learned in part I and II (components in foods and diet/nutrition) to make healthier food choices and allow healthy eating to be part of your lifestyle and not just a diet.
   - You will slowly begin to increase your calories again to a comfortable level not exceeding 1600 calories per day.
   - Once you've mastered the elements to weight loss, you will have weight loss for life.

Exercise Overview

Your exercise training program is very comprehensive. When performed properly and routinely, it will assist you in reaching your weight loss goals, increase endurance, and push your body out of its comfort zone. The program incorporates cardio, calisthenics, interval, flexibility, and weight training and changes with each phase. Make a commitment to yourself and stick to it.

1. **Detox Phase**

   ♦ Cardio at least 30 minutes per day, 5 days per week.

   ♦ Weight training 3 days per week with one exercise per muscle group at a minimum of 15 minutes per day.

   ♦ Flexibility and core training exercises perform simultaneously 3 days per week at a minimum of 20 minutes per day.

   ♦ It is beneficial to add yoga or some other methods of stretching and flexibility to increase the detox process.

2. **Fat Burning Phase**

   ♦ In the fat burning phase, your exercise routine intensifies to allow your body to burn the most calories and fats.

   ♦ Alternating between cardio, calisthenics, and core interval training six days per week. Choose your fitness level and work it.

   ♦ Weight training increase from one exercise per muscle group to two exercises.

   ♦ core and flexibility training Intensify from 20 minutes to 30 minutes three days per week.

3. **Weight Mastery / Healthy 4 Life Phase**

   ♦ Incorporate cardio with interval training six days per week to determine your fitness capabilities.

   ♦ Increase your weight training from two exercises per muscle group to three exercises.

   ♦ Strengthen your core and flexibility training by adding 10 additional minutes of training, 3 days per week.

   Tips to prevent injury and burn out:

   o Start at your fitness level then level up.

o Collaborate with a friend or a fitness coach.
o Always start with a warm-up and end with a cool-down.
o Stretch before and after your workout.
o Do not exercise the same muscle group.
o Choose a program that suits your body type and work with your schedule.
o Take active rest in between sets.
o Wear the proper shoes.

Your Exercise program at a glance!!!

Phases	Cardio	Weight training	Core Flexibility
Phase I Detox	Cardio 30 min/day 5 days/week	1 muscle group 15 min/day 3 days/week	Core 10 min/day Flex 10 min/day 3 days/week
Phase 2 Fat Burning	Interval Training 6 days/week	2 muscle groups 25 min/day 3 days/week	Core 15 min/day Flex 15 min/day 3 days/week
Phase 3 Weight Mastery	Cardio + Interval training 6 days/week	3 muscle groups 35 min/day 3 days/week	Core 20 min/day Flex 20 min/day 3 days/week

Remember *cardio includes brisk walking, jogging, running, cycling, swimming, stair climbing, elliptical trainers, dancing, hiking, etc. Always choose exercises that burn the most calories, challenges your body, and you enjoy fully.*

To maximize on your training program, you should make it a priority to move for 5-10 minutes every hour especially if you have a desk job. Include 5-10 min jumping jacks, jump rope, squats, sit-ups, climbers, or pushups. Any exercise(s) that will increase blood circulation and metabolism and get you moving will be beneficial.

In addition, adhere to the challenges in each phase to maximize on fat loss, increase endurance and stamina, and push your body out of its comfort zone.

Mind-Body Connection Overview

I recommend daily practice of meditation, affirmation, and visualization to foster self-love, self-acceptance, and a more profound connection with your inner self. In addition, journaling, seeking counsel, rest and sleep, play and fun are great tools to incorporate in order to encourage development of a positive body image, balance, and homeostasis. Make a commitment to adhere to the 21-day challenges in each phase they will prove to be extremely beneficial.

Difficulties during the Program

If you encounter difficulties with maintaining the program's regimen, don't give up. Readjust one meal at a time and increase gradually. Grab a friend to do it along with you. Don't stress over it and don't be too hard on yourself. Give it your best shot and stay out of your way.

In addition, don't set your expectations so high that it becomes difficult to achieve your goals. For example, "I want to lose 30lbs in 21-days". Although that is very much achievable, but the stress you will place on your body will cause you to ultimately fail and deem the program ineffective.

Program tasks/challenges

Give yourself a little challenge. Several challenges are added at the end of each phase, to keep you motivated, test your strength and endurance, and enhance the mind-body connection. You will have a diet and nutrition challenge, a physical activity challenge, and a mind-body challenge. Have fun with it and follow through.

Cheating on the program

When people feel restricted, they will find ways to liberate themselves by cheating. Although cheating on any program can surface guilt and a sense of failure, you can allow yourself one day out of the week to enjoy a piece of your favorite snack or to slightly increase your calories without feeling guilty. This will allow you to pacify your cravings and not binge on unhealthy foods such as cakes, cookies, ice cream, and/or potato chips. The key is to *practice self-control, eat in moderation, and keep a continuous vision for success.*

Plan, Plan, Plan

The success of the program depends on proper planning. Many people fail due to lack of planning. Not planning is a recipe 4 failure not a recipe 4 success (R4S). Don't leave anything until last minute.

+ Set up a plan of action for the program.
+ Plan your goals.
+ Plan your meals accordingly.
+ Complete all grocery shopping at the beginning of the week.
+ Separate and bag vegetables and smoothie ingredients for easy access.
+ Keep snacks handy.
+ Schedule mealtime, exercise time, and rejuvenation time (meditation, yoga, journaling, self-work, etc.).
+ Plan, plan, and plan.

Plan, Prepare, and Execute.

Detox Phase

Phase I
Remove the Junk to Jumpstart Weight Loss

Your first 21 days are crucial to the overall success of the program. This phase is designed to jumpstart your weight loss, boost your energy and immunity, remove toxins, fats, and mucus out of your system, heighten your awareness of food allergies, and prepare your body for the subsequent phase.

It is comprised of three important weeks:

1. **Week 1 – Elimination week**
2. **Week 2 – Cleansing week**
3. **Week 3 – Reintroduction week**

Detox Phase - Diet and Nutrition

Daily Meals

- ◆ **Upon rising:** Detox drink and Elixir (water, teas, infused water) or any other detox product(s).

- ◆ **First meal (7am–9 am)**: Your first meal is simple, light, and moderate in size. Your body is still purifying after your night's rest. You can drink a smoothie for your first meal or a protein shake and eat breakfast snack 2-3 hours later. Do not skip your first meal. You're setting the stage for the rest of the day. Skipping breakfast causes food hoarding and overeating later.

- **Second meal (11am–1pm):** Your second meal is largest in calories. You will have ample time to burn off the calories before bed. Keep the calories healthy.
- **Third meal (4pm–7pm):** Your third meal is lowest in calories and carbs (starches, fruits, sugars) and highest in protein. The higher dinner protein facilitates muscle repair, fat burning instead of storing while you're asleep, and better blood sugar balance.
- **1-2 hours after last meal:** Detox drink and elixir (water, teas, infused water.)
- **Snacks:** Keep your snacks healthy and add broth or soups in between meals.

Week 1
Elimination Week

Elimination week is very important so DO NOT attempt to skip it! The elimination week will reduce the extra burden on the digestive organs and prepare the body for cleansing.

Each day you will eliminate certain foods and beverages out of the diet. Foods that cause the most allergies, digestive imbalances, and are more toxic to the liver are eliminated first and reintroduced last. You will keep those foods out of your diet until reintroduction week in week 3. Your diet will be light, clean, and lean with leafy and non-starchy vegetables comprising more than half of your daily meals (60-70%).

How much calories you are consuming is just as important as the type of calories. Leafy and non-starchy vegetables will comprise the bulk of your daily diet, follow by protein, then fat. You may reduce your caloric intake daily until you are consuming less than 1000 calories by day 7 of your elimination week. For instance, if you normally consume 2000 calories per day, begin by decreasing your calories by 150 each day until you reach less than 1000 calories.

By slowly decreasing your calories, you allow your body to:

- Acclimate to the new way of eating,
- Have a smoother transition into cleansing week,
- Prevent your body from going into storage mode,
- Avoid food hoarding and excessive hunger.

Keep in mind that leafy and non-starchy vegetables are high in water and fiber and increasing them in the diet can aid in maintaining satiety. Essential fatty acids derived from fish, fish oils, avocado, nuts, and seeds can keep you satiated. Carry a side salad or celery sticks with almond butter to prevent starvation and overeating between meals.

Your first week sets the foundation for success in the program. Remain true to the elimination week. Follow the suggestions outlined and the meal plans in the "Daily Meal Plan" section. Your determination and triumph will keep you focus on your goals. ***Remember, you're sacrificing one week to gain a lifetime of health; give it your all!***

Day 1

Eliminate all processed foods, soda, hydrogenated oils, alcohol and caffeine containing beverages.

Remove all processed foods out of the diet. In fact, you should utilize the day prior to elimination week to clean out your pantry and refrigerator, as you will not be eating any processed foods for the duration of the program. By getting rid of them, you avoid temptation and can adhere to the diet (out of sight out of mind). Processed foods include boxed goods with added additives, frozen TV dinners, potato chips, fries, and so on.

You will also be eliminating soda, hydrogenated oils, alcohol, and caffeine out of the diet to reduce the toxic burden on your liver and allow it to begin the purging process.

Day 2
Eliminate refined grains and sugars

Refined grains and sugars increase fat build up and cause an array of imbalances. Refined Sugars tend to decrease the immune system and promote inflammation. Diabetes, obesity, and cancer all have been linked to excessive uptake of refined grains and sugars. Remove white flour, white sugar, and white rice out of the diet.

Day 3
Eliminate all dairy products

On day three, you will exclude all dairy products out of the diet including milk, cheese, ice cream, and yogurt. Dairy products are hyper-allergenic, increase mucus production, and can cause unnecessary toxic burden. Furthermore, dairy products can be difficult to digest and people who do not have the enzyme, lactase, to digest milk sugar can exhibit symptoms of lactose intolerant such as bloating, gas, diarrhea, and irritable bowel syndrome. If you fit into that category, choose dairy alternatives instead.

Day 4
Eliminate all red meats

Depending on your overall health, it takes the body 24-72 hours to digest red meat. Removing red meat early out of the diet ensures their complete digestion and excretion out of the colon. In addition, animal products are high in cholesterol, which must be processed by the liver, adding extra body burdens. Red meats include beef, buffalo, goat, lamb, venison, etc.

Day 5
Eliminate all eggs and poultry

Exclude all eggs, chicken, turkey, duck, etc. out of the diet on day 5 to ease the burden on the liver.

Day 6
Eliminate all fish and shellfish

Although fish and shellfish are high in essential fatty acids, removing all seafood prior to your detox week gives your body a break from digesting animal protein. Fish and shellfish include cod, salmon, tilapia, herring, sardines, snapper, scallops, shrimp, etc.

Day 7
Eliminate all grains except sprouted grains

On the final day, eliminate all grains. They are high in calories, dense, and heavy, which can leave you feeling bloated and a little sluggish. Only whole and sprouted grains are allowed.

Week 2
Cleansing Week

Cleansing week is important and essential to weight loss. If this is your first cleanse, day one and two may be a little challenging but stick with it. It is absolutely durable and worth the sacrifice. You will give your body a well-deserved break to facilitate purging of toxins, fats, mucus, and other undesirable residues out of your system through the bowel, urine, sweats, and exhalation.

Why Cleanse?

There is toxicity all around you. The food you eat is often toxic, the water you drink is toxic, and the air you breathe is toxic.

Overloaded toxic materials can accumulate in the fat cells causing obesity, insulin and weight loss resistance by slowing down the metabolic rate, reducing thyroid function, interrupting absorption of crucial vitamins and minerals, down regulating receptor sites for hormones and neurotransmitters, and disrupting pH balance in the gut, blood, and tissues. Furthermore, an increased toxic burden on the body can lead to cancer, inflammation, and skin issues such as acne.

What are the benefits of a good internal cleanse?
A good cleanse when done properly will,
- Increase immune health and circulation,
- Rebalance the organs,
- Rid the body of toxins and excess fats,
- Support the organs of eliminations especially the liver and gallbladder,
- Invite mental clarity,
- Improve digestion and elimination,
- Improve energy and overall appearance (clear skin),
- Increase weight loss,
- Reduce allergies, headaches, joint pain, and sugar cravings,
- Repair any gut dysbiosis,
- Allow your entire body to feel lighter, and
- Enhance overall health.

This is your week to show your strength, self-discipline, and willpower. You can achieve a significant amount of weight loss this week. The diet will be light and clean with plenty of fluid especially water and fiber. There will be no consumption of animal products, grains (unless sprouted), and dairy. You will keep your daily caloric intake at **less than 1000** to allow the digestive organs to function optimally while doing the necessary work to eliminate toxins. You can add cleansing products such as those listed below to facilitate movement of fluids and solids out of the body.

Don't panic *about the calories. Remember leafy vegetables and non-starchy vegetables are low in calories and you can have as much as you desire. You can add 2 tbsp. of olive / flax seed oil per meal or take an omega 3 supplement (fish oil) to keep you satiated.*

The diet will be as follows:

- **Days 1, 2, 6, and 7**

  Consume unlimited amount of fresh leafy and non-starchy vegetables, 3-4 servings of fruits, 2-3 servings of cold-pressed oil (1tbsp/servings), and 1-2 servings of nut butters and sprouted nuts, seeds, and grains.

- **Days 3, 4, and 5**

  You will abstain from eating solids. These will be your liquid only days, smoothies, broths, soups, and water. If you experience symptoms of hypoglycemia, add ¼ cup of brown rice and sprouted nuts.

- **Detox drink**, teas, vitamins, and minerals are all part of the daily diet.

Consider adding:
Herbs:

- Cleansing and supportive herbs: dandelion, milk thistle, burdock root, and red clover
- Cathartic herbs: cascara sagrada, aloe vera, senna, red raspberry, rhubarb
- Expectorant herbs: fenugreek and yarrow

- Parasitic herb: garlic
- Expectorant, anti-inflammatory, cleansing herb: slippery elm bark

Fiber:

- Ground flax seeds,
- Chia seeds,
- Psyllium seed husks, or
- Oat bran

Other:

- Aloe vera juice
- Probiotics (acidophilus or any other strains)
- Super foods: spirulina, chlorella, wheat grass,
- Pancreatic enzymes (twice per day)
- Vitamin C (minimum 1,000mg per day)
- Vitamin E
- Cod liver oil (1000mg per day)
- Activated charcoal
- Purchase a "whole body cleanse" kit from a health food store and use in conjunction with the diet.

Caution: People with severe toxicity or reduced detoxification capacity may experience various symptoms as toxins release into the blood stream.	
If you experience these symptoms:	Do any one or more of these:
Headaches Dizziness Sluggishness Fatigue Skin irritation Muscle aches Constipation	Increase your infused water intake. Increase detox teas. Get an enema or colonic. Add ½ cup of brown rice or rice water to your lunch meal. Keep your body alkaline by increasing consumption of alkaline broth and water. Get a lymphatic massage. Practice deep breathing and/or yoga.

It is important to adhere to the meal plans to ensure a successful cleansing week.

Week 3 - Reintroduction Week

The reintroduction week is your first week following cleansing. You will continue to drink detox teas and detox drinks until the end of this week. It is imperative to reintroduce foods slowly and steadily to avoid food hoarding and overeating.

You will reintroduce foods in the reverse order they were eliminated. For instance, since whole grains were removed last, they will be reintroduced first. Refined grains and sugars, hydrogenated oils, alcoholic beverages, and processed foods will be kept out of the diet for the duration of the program.

You can bypass reintroducing grains in the diet since they will be removed in the fat burning phase or you can add sprouted grains to decrease the heaviness naturally present in grains.

Keep track of your symptoms as you reintroduce hyperallergic foods in the diet. Frequently, following an elimination diet, your body may produce allergic responses such as itching, swelling, bloating, gas, skin rashes, and scratchy throat and palate to certain foods. This means that your body has built-up an intolerance to that food and it's causing your immune system to react. Remove any food(s) that causes such reactions completely out of your diet to decrease inflammation and increase weight loss.

General tips for achieving success in Phase I

If you experience these symptoms:	Try these suggestions:
Constipation	Drink more water. Increase fiber (flax, psyllium husk, slippery elm). Take a magnesium supplement. Get a colonic or enema.

	Add cathartic herbs, vitamin C, vitamin E
Excessive Hunger	Increase EFAs. Eat at a scheduled time. Do not skip meals. Increase water, you may be dehydrated. Add a cup of sprouted grains or beans. Chew, chew, and chew as much as you can before swallowing.
Sugar Cravings	Take a chromium supplement. Increase infused water. Eat a fruit.
Low energy	Drink a shot of wheat grass in the am. Have a cup of green tea or black coffee. Get a B12 shot. Add a multivitamin and a B complex.

Live a toxin free lifestyle

It is not easy to live a toxin free lifestyle as toxicity is all around us daily but we can support the organs of elimination (e.g. bowel, kidneys, liver, lungs, lymphatics, and skin) by following some of the guidelines below:

1. Keep your Bowel moving

The bowel (small and large intestines) is a great organ of elimination. It removes solid waste materials and toxins out of the body. Increasing intake of raw vegetables, leafy greens, fruits, flax seeds, or psyllium husk will reduce the time it takes food wastes to transit through the gut. Dairy products and highly processed foods cause constipation thereby increasing the body's toxic load. Keep them out of the diet as much as possible. Get a colonic or enema to clean your bowel and remove additional toxins.

2. Protect your Kidneys

The kidneys filter out unwanted liquid wastes and play a major role in the cleansing process. Drink a gallon of water per day or a minimum of half your body size in ounces. In addition, you can infuse your water with lemon, peppermint leaves, or cucumber to increase filtration, drink 100% cranberry juice diluted in water to support kidney health, or brew diuretic herbs like dandelion to cleanse the kidneys.

3. Support your Liver

The liver is the main organ of detoxification. It works synergistically with the gallbladder and the other organs of elimination to move toxic material out of the body. To support the liver:

♦ Increase spring vegetables that nourish and support the liver such as dandelion root, burdock root, beet greens, and artichokes.

♦ Limit the intake of alcohol, caffeine, processed foods, preservatives, nicotine, and dyes and exposure to environmental toxins including car exhaust, chemical fumes, and work-related toxic substances, as they cause extra burden on the liver.

♦ Apply castor oil compresses or packs for 45 minutes 2-3 times per week to the liver, located directly below the ribs on the right side of the body.

4. Inhale clean air into your Lungs

The lungs are great organs of detoxification. Practicing deep breathing exercises daily help to keep the lungs clear and the other organs oxygenated. Add aerobic exercises such as running, biking, dancing, jumping, or brisk walking in your daily practice to help the lungs exhale carbon dioxide and inhale more oxygen.

5. Allow continuous lymph and blood circulation

The lymphatic system plays a significant role in transporting lymph, managing fluid levels throughout the body, and filtering out bacteria. Keeping the lymph and blood circulating assure that white blood cells, bacteria, toxins, and other residues are transported to their necessary locations. To support them:

- Engage in daily practice of yoga (preferably hot/bikram yoga), Qi Gong, or Tai Chi, or any other stretching program that increases both blood and lymphatic circulation by releasing muscle constrictions and imbalances.

- Get a lymphatic or regular massage often to improve circulation in the blood and lymphatic system

- Always end a hot shower or bath with a 30-second cold water rinse. This process stimulates the central nervous system and increases circulation.

6. Keep your Skin clear and clean

The skin is your largest organ and serves as a great portal to extract toxin out of the body through the sweat glands. Here are a few things you can do to help your skin with detoxification:

- Skin brushing: skin brushing is a method that aids with lymphatic drainage. Massage your entire body with a dry loofah or natural fiber shower brush (you can find them at any health food store) before getting into the shower or the tub.

- Warm Epsom salt baths: At least once weekly, run a warm water bath, add one to two pounds of Epsom salts (plus one cup sea salt optional), and soak for 20-30 minutes. Drink plenty of water while in the tub and after in order to remain hydrated. You can also drink herbal teas that increase sweating, to sweat out more toxins.

♦ Hygiene: use herbal deodorants instead of antiperspirants to allow the natural flow of sweat to continue the detoxification process. Animal fat soaps and moisturizers tend to clog skin pores, use vegetable oil products instead.

Other things you can do to keep a low toxic burden:

♦ Find ways to destress often

♦ Use the most natural cleaning & cleansing products on yourself and in your home

♦ Avoid plastic bottles and containers that can leach plastic into the food

♦ Use a water and home filter

♦ Take off your shoes at the door to reduce outside chemicals and bacteria

♦ Refrain from using the microwave

Detox Phase: Diet and Nutrition Summary and Recommendations:

☐ Week 1 - Elimination Week
☐ Week 2 - Cleansing Week
☐ Week 3 - Reintroduction Week
☐ Do not skip meals.
☐ Do not overeat or wait too long to eat.
☐ Eat plenty of leafy and non-starchy vegetables.
☐ Drink detox drink and detox teas during the entire phase.
☐ Drink an adequate amount of water each day.
☐ Monitor daily caloric intake, gradually increase to 1200 per day.
☐ Chew, chew, and chew all foods thoroughly.
☐ Do not starve yourself.
☐ Schedule your mealtime wisely.
☐ Do not eat after 7pm or 3 hours before bed.
☐ Add a healthy snack in between meals to maintain a healthy metabolism.
☐ Prepare yourself for fat burning phase.

Detox Phase - Physical Activity

In the first phase of the program, you will begin to incorporate movement again. If you have not exercised in a while, this is the time to grab your workout shoes, dust them off, and start moving. You will include cardio, flexibility, and weight training, at your fitness level.

Start slow, easy, but steady to avoid injuries and burnout. Week 2 is cleansing week, you may feel weak and fatigued, do not overexert yourself. Listen to your body and employ deep breathing exercises or simple yoga moves to allow detoxification to continue.

1. Cardio

Begin by walking or performing any cardiovascular exercise a minimum of 30 minutes per day and 5 days per week. Cardio is not restricted to walking or running, include bicycling, dancing, hiking, or elliptical trainer into your workout. You can increase from 30 minutes to 45 minutes in week 3. *Remember your warm-up and cool down!!!*

2. Weight training

If you are new to weight lifting, begin with one exercise per body part with 3 sets and 8-12 repetitions, resting 60-90 seconds in between sets. If you are at a more advanced level, start with 2 exercises per body part. Start with a weight you can do the most reps with but are fatiguing by the 12th rep.

Warm-up and weight training should precede cardio exercises to prevent injuries and burn the most calories. For instance, if your cardio and weight training are performed in one workout routine, follow the suggestions below:

Time	Exercise
5 min	Warm-up
20-30 min	Weight training

30-45 min	Cardio
5 min	Cool down

3. Core and flexibility

Core and flexibility training should be incorporated in your weekly physical activity.

Your 7-day Beginner Training Program

Week 1, 2, and 3			
Beginner			
Days	**Cardio**	**Strength/Weight training**	**Core and Flexibility**
1	30 min	Upper body - Bicep curls (3 sets, 8-12 reps)	
2	30 min		*5 min abs (2 sets) 10 min Yoga/stretch
3	30 min	Lower Body - Squats (3 sets, 8-12 reps)	
4	10,000 steps		*5 min abs (2 sets) 10 min Yoga/stretch
5	30 min	20 min Deep Breathing	
6	30 min		*5 min abs (2 sets) 10 min Yoga/stretch
7	10,000 steps		

5 min abs = 1 min each of the following exercises with 60 seconds rest in between (crunches, sit-ups, side crunch, leg lifts, plank).

Advanced trainers add an extra upper body and lower body exercise to your routine, perhaps 3 sets of lunges as an adjunct to the squats on day 3 and pushups on day 5.

Detox Phase – Mind-Body Connection

You will need to connect the mind and the body in order to make the detox phase a true success. Change is never easy, but the only thing constant in life is change, subsequently you will adapt. It's "*mind over matter*". By forming a loving relationship with yourself and your body, you can begin to shed more of the undesirable weight. (Read more on the mind/body connection section to remain connected and succeed.)

I emphasized below a few things you can do to enhance the mind-body connection:

- Upon rising, begin with prayer/meditation to set the tone for a successful day.
- Grab your journal and write for 5-15 minutes anything that comes to mind and without judgement.
- Repeat positive affirmative words about yourself while sitting on the bed or standing in front of a mirror.
- Visualize how you would like your body to look and feel.
- Spend time in nature to allow the energy of season to uplift you.
- Set time to write down your daily and weekly goals.
- Foster a positive attitude towards food.
- Get plenty of rest and adequate amount of sleep.
- Keep calm and away from arguments, your body functions best when it is not in a constant state of "fight or flight".
- Partake in fun activities.
- Set your mind up for success.

Detox Phase – Challenges

These are your first 21-day diet & nutrition, exercise, and mind/body challenges. Print them and post them on your wall or refrigerator door for easy access. Attempt at accomplishing each one daily and be easy on yourself if you skip a day or two.

Detox Phase - Diet and Nutrition Challenge

Your challenge is to drink as much water as possible to flush out toxins, hydrate your organs, and reach 1 gallon of water on day 21. You can also maintain the daily recommendation of half of your body weight in ounces. As long as you drink an adequate amount of water daily, you enhance the detoxification process and accelerate weight loss.

In addition, if you prefer flavored water, infuse your water with slices of lemon, lime, orange, ginger, or cucumber. Mint leaves are diuretic and add great flavor to the water. This process also boosts detoxification through the kidneys by increasing water excretion. *Do not substitute water for Gatorade, store bought flavored water, crystal lite, etc. simply pure natural water or infused water.*

Water Challenge						
1 56 oz.	2 56 oz.	3 64 oz.	4 64 oz.	5 64 oz.	6 72 oz.	7 72 oz.
8 80 oz.	9 80 oz.	10 88 oz.	11 88 oz.	12 96 oz.	13 96 oz.	14 104 oz.
15 104 oz.	16 112 oz.	17 112 oz.	18 120 oz.	19 120 oz.	20 128 oz.	21 128 oz.

Detox Phase - Physical Activity Challenge

This is a great phase to begin incorporating yoga daily. If you are new to yoga, read more about it, join a yoga class, checkout a video from the library, or watch it online. Yoga increases flexibility while fostering a deeper self-connection and awareness.

Yoga Challenge						
1 10 min yoga	2 10 min yoga	3 10 min yoga	4 15 min yoga	5 15 min yoga	6 15 min yoga	7 20 min yoga
8 20 min yoga	9 20 min yoga	10 25 min yoga	11 25 min yoga	12 25 min yoga	13 30 min yoga	14 30 min yoga
15 30 min yoga	16 35 min yoga	17 35 min yoga	18 40 min yoga	19 40 min yoga	20 45 min yoga	21 45 min yoga

You may substitute yoga for Pilates, Qi Gong, or any other flexibility training.

Detox Phase - Mind/Body Challenge

Your mind/body challenge is to incorporate meditation and journaling as a daily practice for at least 21 days. The benefits you attain may drive you towards maintaining a regular practice. In your meditation, include mantras and deep breathing work. In your journaling, write affirmations, goals, aspirations, triggers, likes and dislikes, and areas for self-improvements. Describe vividly and with emotions your dream or perfect body.

Meditation & Journal Challenge						
1 5min M 4 min J	2 5min M 5 min J	3 5min M 6 min J	4 10min M 7 min J	5 10min M 8 min J	6 10min M 9 min J	7 15min M 10 min J
8 15min M 10 min J	9 15min M 10 min J	10 15min M 11 min J	11 15min M 12 min J	12 15min M 14 min J	13 20min M 15 min J	14 20min M 15 min J
15 20min M 15 min J	16 25min M 16 min J	17 25min M 17 min J	18 25min M 18 min J	19 30min M 19 min J	20 30min M 20 min J	21 30min M 20 min J

*Meditation (M) * Journal (J)*

Fat Burning Phase

Phase II
Maximizing on Fat Loss

The fat burning phase requires discipline and self-control. It allows you to maximize on fat loss, increase metabolism, and burn the most calories to lead you closer to your ideal weight. If this phase is done correctly, you will lose the most weight and be well on your way to attaining success.

You may continue this phase until you achieve weight loss goal or alternate between this phase and the weight mastery phase every 21 days.

Fat Burning Phase - Diet and Nutrition

Daily Meals

- Prior to first meal, drink 10 ounces of warm lemon infused water or pure water.

- **First meal (7am–9 am):** Your first meal is comprised of a protein shake. You may eat a high protein breakfast with leafy vegetables and some good fats. For example, you can have scrambled eggs with spinach. You should also drink enough water to enhance the purification process 10 minutes before and after your meal.

  You are allowed 20g of carbohydrates with your protein shake. Weigh and count your carbs.

Eat within 30 minutes to 1 hour of exercising in the morning. You can add a pre- and post- workout protein shake.

♦ **Second meal (11am–1pm):** Your second meal is largest in calories and carbs. It should contain 30g of leafy and non-starchy vegetables, 4 ounces of protein, and 4 tbsp. of fat. Count your carbs; they should not exceed 30g.

♦ **Third meal (4pm – 7pm):** Your third meal is lowest in carbs but highest in protein. The higher dinner protein facilitates muscle repair and regeneration of muscle fibers, fat burning instead of storing while you're asleep, and better blood sugar balance.

Your dinner meal should contain 6 ounces of lean protein, 2-3 servings of fat, and about 20g of leafy/non-starchy vegetables.

♦ No food after 7pm or 3 hours before bed. If exercising after dinner, add a protein shake.

♦ **Snacks**: All snacks should contain no more than 7g of carbs.

As you learned from the previous sections, carbohydrates are the main source of fuel utilized by the body. When they are in excess, the body stores them as fat in the form of triglycerides. During the fat burning phase, you will allow your body to tap into its reserved fats and utilize those as fuel by switching from carbohydrate breakdown into glucose to fat metabolism.

The diet will consist of healthy fats, adequate amount of lean protein, leafy and non-starchy vegetables, and plenty of infused water.

How much protein, carbohydrate, and fat should you consume per meal?

For this phase of the program, concentrate on counting your carbs and keeping them as low as possible. Carbohydrates will be restricted to about 50-60g per day of leafy and non-starchy vegetables and 10g of fruits. Only eat fruits in the morning, add to protein shake or smoothie.

Fats (60%) will comprise a major portion of your daily meals follow by protein (30%) then carbs (10%). Your protein will be lean and your fats will include cold-pressed oils, nuts, and seeds, avocado, and coconut oil.

All starchy vegetables are eliminated to allow the body to break down fat and utilize fat metabolism as fuel. All boxed and processed foods should be removed as well.

You will consume approximately:
- *4-6oz of lean and clean protein per meal,*
- *50-60g of leafy and non-starchy vegetables and 10g of fruits per day, and*
- *4 or more servings of fat per meal.*

How will you shift your metabolism and burn more fat?

There are many studies and diet books in the market and their approaches differ tremendously. The bottom line is, in order to shift your metabolism and burn more fat:

- You must **change** the way you eat and how much you eat.
- You need an **adequate amount of protein** in the diet. Protein can increase your metabolic rate by as much as 30%, build and maintain lean muscle mass, and increase weight loss.
- You must **reduce the amount of carbohydrates** that you take in per meal.
- You must **remain hydrated**.
- You may have to eat at a **scheduled time** because when the body is aware that food is on the way, it speeds up metabolism.

- **You cannot skip meals or overeat**. Skipping meals slow down your metabolism and cause you to eat more at the next meal. Overeating increases fat storage.
- You must **change the old habits** that were not beneficial in the past and welcome new ones.
- You **CANNOT STARVE** yourself. Starvation does not work. You must eat enough not to cause your body to experience starvation. The latter decreases metabolism and causes food hoarding / overeating, which inhibits weight loss.
- You must include exercise as part of your daily routine.

What's an acceptable caloric intake that will shift your body into fat loss?

Since fats are high in calories, they will cover the majority of your calories. Protein will be the next high calorie nutrient. Carbohydrates will take up less of the calories (about 10-15%) since you will consume mainly leafy green, raw, and non-starchy vegetables high in water and fiber. Watch out for hidden carbohydrates in salad dressings and condiments. Make your own salad dressings at the beginning of the week for easy accessibility.

Keep your calories at an adequate amount. I recommend between 1000 and 1600. Increase to the higher end only if you challenge your body with physical activity and you are consuming essential fatty acids (EFA).

General tips for the Fat Burning Phase:

If you experience these symptoms:	Try these suggestions:
Slight constipation	Drink more water. Increase fiber (flax, psyllium husk, slippery elm).

	Take a magnesium supplement. Get a colonic or enema. No laxatives
Increased Urination	Take a potassium supplement to replace potassium loss.
Excessive Hunger	Increase EFAs. Eat at a scheduled time. Do not skip meals. Increase water, you may be dehydrated.
Cravings	Take a chromium supplement. Increase infused water.
Low energy	Drink a shot size of wheat grass in the am. Have a cup of green tea or black coffee. Get a B12 shot. Add a multivitamin and a B complex.

Fat Burning Phase: Diet and Nutrition Summary and Recommendations

❑ Increase infused water intake, essential fatty acids, and lean protein.

❑ Reduce carbs – 50–60g per day leafy greens and non–starchy vegetables only and 10g fruits.

❑ Keep all grains, sweeteners, fried foods, processed foods, and alcohol out of the diet.

❑ No food after 7 pm or 3 hours before bed.

❑ If you exercise after 7pm, have a high protein snack or drink a protein shake.

❑ Purchase a high quality protein powder with 20–30g of protein per serving and 0–3g of carbs. You can purchase whey protein or vegetarian/vegan protein powder without grains, try hemp, pea protein, or chia seed protein.

❑ Add a 1000mg cod liver oil or flax seed oil per day.

❑ Add supplements that increase fat loss such as CLA, L–carnitine, or Garcinia Cambodia (see Supplements section in Part I).

❑ Drink green tea, black coffee, or a shot of wheat grass juice before exercise to boost energy and burn more calories.

❑ Do not skip your any meals.

❑ Add a snack in between to speed up metabolism.

Fat Burning Phase - Physical Activity

Your second phase physical activity is all about challenging your body to burn the most fat in 21 days.

1. Cardio

Your cardio will comprise of interval training, a minimum of 6 days per week, 20-30 minutes per day, and preferably in the morning. A day of high intensity interval training (HIIT) will follow with a less intense day of cardio interval training, which will allow your body to recuperate.

If you are bypassing interval training and are sticking to regular cardio, increase your cardio from 30 minutes to 45 minutes per day, 6 days per week. You can always substitute jogging/running for bicycling, swimming, or elliptical trainer. The latter exercises remove pressure on your knee joints and improve performance. ***Remember your warm-up and cool down!!!***

2. Weight training

Beginners increase from 1 exercise per body part to 2 exercises with 3 sets and 8-12 repetitions, resting 60-90 seconds in between sets. Again, start with a weight you can do the most reps with but are fatiguing by the 12th rep. ***Remember warm-up and weight training should precede cardio exercises.***

Time	Exercise
5 min	Warm-up
20-30 min	Weight training
30-45 min	Cardio
5 min	Cool down

3. Core and Flexibility

Incorporate core and flexibility exercises a minimum of 3 days per week. Flexibility should always follow every warm-up and cool down to prevent soreness. To increase flexibility and agility, I suggest 3 days of flexibility training. Your core exercises will be HIIT 4 varying between 15 seconds and 1 minute training, 4 days a week.

Week 4, 5, and 6			
Beginner			
Days	Cardio	Strength/Weight training	Core & Flexibility
1	15 sec HIIT 1 (week 4) 15 sec HIIT 2 (week 5) 15 sec HIIT 3 (week 6)		15 sec HIIT 4 15 min yoga/stretch
2	Cardio interval training 20-30 minutes	Upper body **Biceps** (3 sets, 8-12 reps)	
3	20 sec HIIT 1 (week 4) 20 sec HIIT 2 (week 5) 20 sec HIIT 3 (week 6)		20 sec HIIT 4 15 min yoga/stretch
4	10, 000 steps	Lower Body **Barbell Squats** & **Calf raises** (3 sets, 8-12 reps)	
5	30 sec HIIT 1 (week 4) 30 sec HIIT 2 (week 5) 30 sec HIIT 3 (week 6)		30 sec HIIT 4 15 min yoga/stretch
6	Cardio interval training 20-30 minutes	Upper body **Bench press** (3 sets, 8-12 reps)	
7	1 min HIIT 1 (week 4) 1 min HIIT 2 (week 5) 1 min HIIT 3 (week 6)		1 min HIIT 4 15 min yoga /stretch

Fat Burning Phase – Mind-Body

The fat burning phase requires discipline and self-confidence. It will test your willpower and ability to follow through and adhere to change. Continue to foster that mind-body connection to make this phase a true success. Your challenge is to state daily affirmations along with visualization to accelerate weight loss progress.

Quick Reminders!!!

♦ Begin your day with prayer/meditation/affirmation to realign your thoughts and set the tone for the rest of the day

♦ Grab your journal and write for 5-15 minutes anything that comes to mind and without judgement.

♦ Focus on this phase's mind-body challenge to visualize your ideal body.

♦ Foster a positive attitude towards food and eating.

♦ Be easy on yourself.

♦ Reward yourself for a job well done.

♦ Get plenty of rest and adequate amount of sleep.

♦ Set your mind up for success.

Fat Burning Phase Challenges

Use this phase challenges to keep you motivated, push your body to the next level, and envision that perfect body.

Fat Burning Phase - Diet and Nutrition Challenge

You will have a **No Sugar Challenge** to allow your body to burn reserved fat efficiently. You can have **one fruit** in the morning. Table sugar, milk chocolate, pastries, cakes, sweeteners (natural and artificial) are not allowed. It's only 21 days, you can do it!!!
If sugar is not your weakness, replace it with your favorite unhealthy snacks or alcohol.

No Sugar Challenge						
No sugar No chocolate No sweeteners						
1	2	3	4	5	6	7
Challenge is on, I'm ready	This is easy	I got this under control!	Who said I couldn't do it	Mind over matter	It's not the end of the world	Yes, one week down. Yeah me!!!
8	9	10	11	12	13	14
I am strong	Let see, only 1, 2, 3, ... Ummmm I can do it!	I can achieve my goal faster	I am a champion!	I turn my head and say "not today"	I got this!	Only one week left
15	16	17	18	19	20	21
Two weeks down ... one to go I got it!	Hang tight!	I am a winner @ everything.	I am so close	Only two more days	I'm almost there	I did it!!! Time to celebrate with more exercise

Fat Burning Phase - Physical Activity Challenge

Squats strengthen and build muscle mass in the lower body and core. They improve flexibility, help burn fat more efficiently, and increase release of testosterone and growth hormones. In the fat burning phase challenge, you will test your strength by increasing the amount of squats by 25 every week. It is a gradual increase so you can do it.

Squats Challenge						
1 10 RS 5 PS	2 10 RS 5 JS	3 15 RS 10 PS 5 JS	4 15 RS 30 sec WS	5 20 RS 15 PS 10 JS	6 20 RS 30 sec WS	7 50 squats
8 25 RS 15 PS 10 JS	9 25 RS 45 sec WS	10 30 RS 20 PS 15 JS	11 30 R 20 P 15 J	12 35 RS 45 sec WS	13 35 RS 25 PS 15 JS	14 75 squats
15 40 RS 1 min WS	16 40 RS 30 JS	17 45 RS 35 PS	18 45 RS 1 min WS	19 50 RS 25 PS 20 JS	20 50 RS 25 PS 25 JS	21 100 squats

RS = Regular Squats ♦ PS = Plier Squats ♦ JS = Jump Squats ♦ WS = Wall Squats

You have the option to utilize weights such as dumbbells with your squats. Adding weights will enhance the challenge, help burn more calories, and strengthen both upper and lower body.

Fat Burning Phase – Mind-Body Challenge

Your challenge is to state **affirmations** for the next 21 days while utilizing **visualization** and emotions as your guides. For example, when you state "I am skinny", close your eyes and imagine what skinny looks like to you, feel it, be it, and see it, as it has already manifested.

Affirmations/Visualization Challenge						
1 I am perfect	2 I am healthy	3 I am happy	4 I am fit	5 I am energized	6 I am wonderfully made	7 I am beautiful inside and out
8 My body is flawless	9 My body is healthy	10 My body is stunning	11 My body is strong	12 My body is responsive to healthy eating	13 My body is on point	14 I love my body and my body loves me
15 I love myself	16 I am pleased with my body	17 I love who I am becoming	18 I am irresistible	19 I am skinny	20 I fit into my favorite swimsuit	21 I achieve my goal weight

You can replace any phrase(s) for words that fit you best. Remain true to the process and have fun with it. It will accelerate weight loss.

Weight Mastery / Healthy 4 Life Phase

Phase III

Setting the stage
4 continuous weight loss success

Weight Mastery is your final 21-day phase. You removed the junk in phase I. You maximized on fat loss in phase II. Phase III allows you to master your weight and remain healthy 4 life by putting into practice your R4S.

You can alternate between this phase and the fat burning phase until you reach your weight loss goals.

How can you incorporate R4S beyond the program?

Incorporating the three components of R4S will be of utmost importance as you continue on your weight loss journey:

1) **Healthy Eating (HE)** which include Adequate Caloric Intake (ACI) and Portion Control (PC)
2) **Exercise (E)**, and
3) **Mind-Body Connection (MBC)**

They each play fundamental roles in achieving sustainable weight loss. When all factors add up, you have a true **recipe for success (R4S)**.

$$HE + E + PA = (R4S)$$

1. Healthy Eating (HE)

The first component of R4S is vital not only to weight loss but to overall health and wellness as well. 75-80% of weight loss is attributed to healthy eating and making healthy choices. If you make it a lifestyle, overtime your body will function at an optimal level, you will maintain a healthy body weight, and you will decrease risk of preventable illnesses such as diabetes and high blood pressure.

ACI and PC are two major parts of HE that will play key roles in weight mastery as you start to make healthier choices.

Adequate Caloric Intake (ACI)

Caloric intake has been an ongoing debate among weight loss experts. Some believe that calories are not important as long as you control your portion size. Others argue that it is crucial to weight loss and must remain low to reach weight mastery. Which is the correct argument?

I believe daily caloric intake must be included in the weight loss puzzle. After all, we don't become obese from adequate consumption of calories. Furthermore, we have been programmed to believe that our bodies need a significant amount of calories for survival when in fact the body functions best with lower calories at a higher nutritional content. The body's demand for more is frequently caused by:

- Dehydration
- Malnutrition
- Stress and stressors
- Emotional and Hormonal imbalances
- Nutritional depletion of vital nutrients

The dietary guidelines change to conform to new ways of eating. A few decades ago, a daily caloric intake of less than 1000 calories was more than enough to fulfill the body's needs and demands. Added chemicals to our foods, which manipulate the brain responses, lead to cravings, overeating, and excessive caloric intake.

A diet high in calories especially from unhealthy and processed foods such as potato chips, cakes, pizza, pies, burgers, and fries causes the body to store fat instead of breaking it down, rob the body of essential nutrients, and increase fat production.

There are various tools available both electronic and paper format to assist with calorie counting and tracking of food intake. You can also purchase and download "*The Perfect 60-Day Diet and Exercise companion*", to keep track of your progress. Research has shown that people who keep track of their food intake and exercise routines are more likely to be successful and tend to reach their weight loss goals faster than those who do not.

Q and A (Q=Questions A=Answers)

Q: Should I continue to monitor my calories if I exercise?

A: Yes. If your goal is weight loss, exercise will not get you where you need to be if 1) your daily caloric intake super exceeds your caloric output and 2) your diet is high in fast and processed foods. Your calories should be at a reasonable range to allow continuous fat loss and maintenance once you've achieved your weight loss goal.

Q: How much calories should I consume?

A: For long-term weight loss, a daily caloric intake that does not surpass 1600 calories should be suitable as long as exercise is part of the daily routine otherwise maintain your daily intake between 1000 and 1400 calories. Caloric content should be from high fiber vegetables, fruits, essential fatty acids, and lean protein. You will notice as you begin to count calories that fats and simple carbs increase net calories. Monitor your total fat and carbohydrates intake in the diet. Once you adhere to consuming essential fatty acids and more leafy and non-starchy vegetables, your calories will remain at an adequate level for weight loss and maintenance.

Q: Will I lose the weight faster if I starve myself?

A: A low caloric intake does not equate to starvation. You have to eat enough to maintain a healthy metabolism while not overeating. Starvation decreases metabolism and leads to food hoarding, fat storage, muscle wasting, and blood sugar irregularities. To lose sustainable weight, you must make healthy choices and eat an adequate amount of calories per meals.

Portion Control (PC)

Portion control has been a debatable issue as well. It is imperative to control your portion size regardless of whether you're eating well or not. The higher your portion size the higher the calories, unless it's a large bowl of salad with no dressings.

A properly portioned plate for weight mastery should contain 3-4 ounces of protein the size of one's palm (about 30% of the plate), a side of leafy greens, and a side of non-starchy vegetables (about 70% of the plate). Fruits, starches, grains, and beans can be added at the end of the meal or eaten as separate meals or snacks whenever possible since they alter protein digestion.

2. Exercise

While exercise only comprises 20% of weight loss, it is a major component of R4S for the reasons stated in the physical activity section and needs to be incorporated daily.

Q: Can I substitute exercise for eating healthy?

A: Absolutely NOT.

This happens to most of us. Once we begin to exercise regularly, we think it's ok to give ourselves a free pass or reward ourselves with junk foods or high calorie meals. We substitute exercise for healthy eating hoping that exercise will take care of the extra calories. Although this may work in certain cases, military training for instance, it does not work for long-term sustainable weight loss.

Let's do a little math. Suppose you've already consumed 1500 calories prior to your workout. You go to the gym and burn 500 calories during an intense workout routine. To reward yourself you eat a heavy fatty meal with desert, equaling approximately 1000 calories (on the low side). Your total calories consumption for the day is now 2500 calories. Once you subtract the 500 calories you burned, you're left with 2000 calories.

2500 (input) – 500 (output) = 2000 (Net calories)

You have a positive net caloric intake of 2000 calories. Guess where the excess calories end up? That's right, **fat storage**. Your brain only needs a limited amount of glucose to function and your muscles unless you're actively doing work, will not utilize that much fuel. The remainder of the calories will be stored as fat for later use. Yes, it's true that you do burn calories, breathing, talking, sitting, and even sleeping, but not enough to prevent weight gain.

In practicing such method, you will retain your current weight or lose it at a much slower rate. Overtime, you will give up on your weight loss goals due to lack of results. For successful weight loss, diet and exercise go hand in hand; one should not replace the other.

Unhealthy eating should never be your reward after exercise. In fact, you should utilize your post workout meal(s) to replenish your muscles and tissues. During any exercise routine, you are breaking down muscle fibers and many other components in your body. Your post workout should contain adequate amount of protein, good fats, and healthy carbs to support the body in repair and maintenance.

Furthermore, in weight loss, your priorities are nutrition and negative net caloric intake at the end of the day.

Calorie in = calorie out

Proper diet and exercise lead to immediate success.

3. Mind-Body Connection

The last piece of R4S is fostering a mind-body connection and keeping a positive attitude. When we foster a positive attitude about anything in life, goodness flows naturally. As it pertains to weight loss, keeping a positive attitude towards foods, body image, and the way you feel about yourself and others continuously lead to that mind-body connection, self-love, and weight loss. (Read more on this in the mind/body connection section).

Weight Mastery Phase - Diet and Nutrition

In this phase, your meals reflect how you should eat beyond the program to facilitate weight mastery and to remain healthy 4 life. Keep your meals simple, easy, and under 30-minute prep time. Add variety to decrease boredom. Eat locally and seasonally grown foods, they are more nutritious and lower in pesticides.

Your Daily Meals:

- Always start with 10 ounces of warm infused water to clean your system.
- **First meal (7am–9 am):** Your first meal can include a smoothie, protein shake, or a light and healthy breakfast with plenty of fluid before and after your meal.

- **Second meal (11am–1pm):** Your second meal should be largest in calories. You have plenty of time to burn them off before bed. You can include 1-2 servings of starches high in fiber such as sprouted quinoa or brown rice, sweet potatoes in the fall, or summer and winter squashes.

- **Third meal (4pm–7pm):** Your third meal will be lowest in carbs. You dinner meal should contain 50g of carbs or less. Maintain protein at 4-5oz.

- Do not eat after 7 pm or 3 hours before bed. Drink a protein shake or eat a high protein snack if you exercise after 7pm.

- Once a week, two animal protein meals are substituted for two plant-based meals to alleviate digestive load, increase fiber in the diet, and maintain health.

Diet and Nutrition Recommendations for weight mastery:

- ❑ Starches should remain sprouted and limited in the diet until you reach your weight loss goal.
- ❑ Processed foods, soda, hydrogenated oils, and alcohol should be eaten sparingly. Designate one day out of the week to consume them, if you must have them.
- ❑ Do not restrict yourself too much but monitor your calories and portion sizes
- ❑ Eat at a scheduled time to ovoid overeating or sugar cravings.
- ❑ Maintain a healthy daily regimen by continuing to add salad as a main or a side dish.
- ❑ Eat a variety of locally grown and seasonal vegetables.
- ❑ Carry a fruit and some nuts with you at all times for quick snack when you feel hungry.
- ❑ Do not skip meals.
- ❑ Do not overeat or wait too long to eat.
- ❑ Do not starve yourself.
- ❑ The key is moderation.

Weight Mastery - Physical Activity

You're building up from the fat burning phase to adapt to a routine that suits your schedule and body type. You can change your routine every 3 weeks to prevent plateau and increase endurance and physical fitness.

1. Cardio

You will be alternating between regular cardio 30-45 minutes per day and interval training 6 days per week. The goal is to maintain an exercise routine that is constantly challenging your body. Add some fun physical activities such as hiking, biking, swimming dancing, or join a team or boot camp. ***Remember your warm-up and cool down!!!***

2. Weight training

You will increase from two exercises per body part to three exercises while maintaining the same number of sets, repetitions, and rest time (3 sets and 8-12 repetitions resting 60-90 seconds in between sets). Increase your weight to one you can do the most reps with but are fatiguing by the 12th rep. You should dedicate at least 30 minutes to weight training with a minimum of 3 days per week. ***Remember to add a warm-up and a cool-down, and weight training should precede cardio workouts.***

Time	Exercise
5 min	Warm-up
20-30 min	Weight training
30-45 min	Cardio
5 min	Cool down

3. Core and Flexibility

It is important to continue a core and flexibility regimen in this phase and beyond the nine weeks because of all the benefits that they both provide. You can always incorporate time for core and flexibility before and after your cardio or following strength training. I do recommend a minimum of 3 days per week, 20-30 minutes per day.

You can follow this program or any program that suits you best.

Week 7, 8, and 9			
Beginner			
Days	Cardio	Strength/Weight training	Core & Flexibility
1	Cardio 30-45 min	Upper body (3 sets, 8-12 reps) **Biceps and Back** Bicep curls Hammer curls Back extensions	
2	Interval Training		40 min
3	Cardio 30-45 min	Lower Body (3 sets, 8-12 reps) **Legs** Leg curls Leg extensions Calf raises	
4	Interval Training		40 min
5	Cardio 30-45 min	Upper body (3 sets, 8-12 reps) **Triceps & Chest** Triceps dips Bench press Pushups	
6	Interval Training		40 min
7	Rest	Rest	Rest

Weight Mastery – Mind-Body Connection

The mind-body component is as important in this last phase as the other two phases. Continual self-love, affirmations, meditation, and self-work are warranted. Follow the guidelines outlined in the mind-body component section to adhere to a regimen that will yield success. In addition, remember to:

- State affirmations and meditate daily.
- Visualize your ideal body weight daily.
- Make a commitment to write thoughts, ideas, and plans in a notebook or journal.
- Join a boot camp, a fitness club, or a hiking group to keep you motivated and focus on your goals.
- Spend time outside.
- Foster a positive attitude towards food and eating.
- Get plenty of rest and adequate amount of sleep.
- Keep calm and away from arguments, your body functions best when it is not in a constant state of "*fight or flight*".
- Partake in fun activities with family and friends.
- Set your mind up for continual success.

Weight Mastery - Challenges

Weight Mastery Phase - Diet & Nutrition Challenge

In the next 21 days, you will incorporate various diet and nutrition challenges in your daily routine as a reminder to eat well and stay healthy.

Stay Well! Challenge						
1 Eat a healthy breakfast	2 Enjoy a side salad	3 Stop eating by 7pm	4 Include plenty of leafy greens	5 Eat in moderation	6 Drink plenty of H_2O	7 Juice
8 Try a vegetarian dish	9 Make healthy choices	10 Drink plenty of H_2O	11 Include a variety of seasonal vegetables	12 Count your calories	13 Treat yourself to some dark chocolate	14 Sprout your beans & add them to salads
15 Sprout your grains	16 Enjoy a handful of fresh berries	17 No starches after 4pm	18 Drink a Smoothie	19 Dedicate 30 min to sit and enjoy your meal.	20 Eat a healthy snack	21 Juice

You can substitute your own.

Weight Mastery Phase - Exercise Challenge

The exercise challenge of this last phase, challenges your strength, endurance, and willpower. You will begin with 100 reps and increase by 100 each week. Split your exercise into sets or spread them throughout the day, if that will work best for you and your schedule.

For instance,

- Divide your day's reps into 5 sets with 30 seconds to 1-minute rest in between. 100 squats = 5 sets with 20 reps.

- Spread your workout throughout the day: 25 before breakfast, 25 in the afternoon, 25 before dinner, and 25 a couple of hours before bed.

- To make it a true challenge do as fewer sets as possible.

The Big 100 Challenge						
1 100 Jump rope Skips	2 100 Squats	3 100 Jumping Jacks	4 100 Crunches	5 100 High knees	6 100 Pushups	7 100 Leg lifts
8 200 Jump rope Skips	9 200 Squats	10 200 Jumping Jacks	11 200 Crunches	12 200 High knees	13 200 Pushups	14 200 Leg lifts
15 300 Jump rope Skips	16 300 Squats	17 300 Jumping Jacks	18 300 Crunches	19 300 High knees	20 300 Pushups	21 300 Leg lifts

Weight Mastery Phase – Mind-Body Challenge

This is the last phase of the program and it's time to reward yourself for all your hard work. Your challenge is to pamper yourself everyday by doing something that makes you happy and warms your heart. I have included some suggestions below. You can always add your own. Try not to reward yourself with junk or unhealthy foods.

Pamper Yourself Challenge						
1 Get a massage	2 Take a warm bath	3 Spend time outside	4 Connect with a friend	5 Go out dancing	6 Get a pedicure	7 Do something outside the norm
8 Sing in the shower	9 Meditate for 20 min or more	10 Go on a day retreat	11 Listen to music	12 Take a nap in the middle of the day	13 Get a manicure	14 Go hiking
15 Go out on a date	16 Have a spa day	17 Take a "me" day	18 Laugh for no reason	19 Take up yoga	20 Achieve 1 thing from your bucket list	21 Journal for 20 minutes

Daily Meal Plans

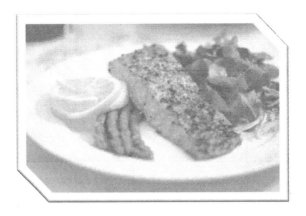

✿✿✿

H aving pre-set daily meal plans add to the recipe for success. Your only task is to lay a plan of action in motion, write your grocery shopping list for the week, and gear your mind for success.

General Overview of all meals

- ◆ Your meals are light, colorful, clean, and lean to encourage weight loss and healthy.
- ◆ Seasonal harvests are included in daily meals (check the area where you reside for substitution).
- ◆ Both sea and land proteins are utilized in the diet (keep in mind that you can substitute any protein as long as you keep it lean).
- ◆ Fruits and starches such as grains and yams can be an added snack in between your meals and are only included in the last phase.
- ◆ Water is part of the daily nutrient and is included in the daily meal plan.

Reminders:

- ◆ *There are no starches after 4 pm and all meals should end by 7 pm or 3 hours before bed to disallow food to sit in your stomach while you're sleeping.*
- ◆ *Drink a morning elixir soon after rising (see examples of morning elixirs in the recipe section) to support and continue purification.*
- ◆ *Morning cardio tap into your stored fat and should be done prior to eating breakfast.*
- ◆ *Use clean and healthy snacks in between meals. You can break your 3 meals into six smaller meals or add a protein shake in between. Add broth as a snack.*
- ◆ *Eat at the first sign of hunger.*

- *Do not wait too long to eat.*
- *Do not overeat.*
- *Drink plenty of water in between meals and use my rule of 10 before and after meals.*
- *Use the recipes at the end of the book for daily meals.*
- ***Your order of eating: 1) proteins, 2) nuts and oils, 3) starches, 4) vegetables, 5) fruits, 6) desserts***

Shopping Tips:

- *Shop with a grocery list.*
- *Make your grocery list based on the weekly menus.*
- *Shop often for fresh produce.*
- *Shop with all your senses.*
- *Shop the perimeter of the grocery store.*
- *Do not shop on an empty stomach.*
- *Do not substitute value for price and vice versa.*
- *Visit a health food store if you are unable to find organic foods at your local grocery store.*

Meal Prep Tips:

- *Individually bag the week's smoothie ingredients small Ziploc bag for each day.*
- *Wash and bag all ingredients for stir-fry, kabobs, or roasted/grilled vegetables in separate Ziploc bags and label.*
- *Prepare and cook most of your protein at the beginning of each week by following the recipes outlined in the recipe section.*
- *Separate your cooked proteins into 3-6 ounces and store in the refrigerator.*

- *Make up a week's worth of salad and vinaigrette and store separately in the refrigerator.*
- *If eating out, remember what's allowed and what's not.*
- *Weigh all proteins cooked and all vegetables raw.*

Detox Phase Brief Recap!!!

	Fat Burning Phase	*Challenges*
Diet & Nutrition	*Week 1 – Elimination* *Week 2 – Cleansing* *Week 3 – Reintroduction* *Monitor caloric intake*	**Water Challenge** *1 gallon by day 21* *Or* *Half your body weight in ounces everyday*
Exercise	*Cardio: 30 min – 5 days per week.* *Strength: 20 minutes* *Core: 10 minutes* *Flexibility: 10 minutes*	**Yoga challenge** *45 min by day 21*
Mind-Body	*Affirmation / Meditation / Journal / Visualization / Self-work*	**Meditation / Journal** *30 min Meditation* *20 min Journal* *(by day 21)*

Remember:

- ♦ *No food after 7 pm or 3 hours before bed*
- ♦ *Keep carbs between 100-120 grams (g) per day.*
- ♦ *Monitor daily caloric intake.*
- ♦ *You can substitute morning smoothie for healthy breakfast as long as you increase water consumption.*
- ♦ *Check recipes in the Recipe section for daily meals.*

Are you ready for your first successful 21 days? Well, I am, so come on!!!

Snacks

Snacks can be added in between meals to maintain metabolism. Only healthy snacks are allowed. Do not snack on potato chips, sugary sweets like cookies, or nutritionally depleted products. Keep your snacks within 100-200 calories. If you drink a smoothie in the morning, add a breakfast snack 2-3 hours later. Nuts are high in fats and calories, do not overconsume.

Snacks should follow the guidelines for each week. For instance, on day 5 of elimination week, you are eliminating all eggs. Hence, you wouldn't include eggs as snacks.

Your snack and breakfast options include:

- 2-3 hard boil eggs with 2 slices of tomatoes
- 5 egg whites scrambled with spinach
- 3-4 nitrite free turkey bacon with side steamed vegetables
- Turkey sausage with sautéed vegetables
- Oatmeal with berries and walnuts
- Tofu scramble with spinach
- Chia seeds pudding parfait
- Celery sticks with almond butter
- 10-15 almonds with 3-4 strawberries
- Small side salad with protein
- Seaweed salad
- 1-2 cups of soup
- Broths (alkaline/immune broths)

Week 1 – Elimination Week

Day	Breakfast	Lunch	Dinner
1	Smoothie Multivitamin	**Chicken kabobs + cauliflower rice** Chicken Mixed Vegetables Cauliflower	**Tossed grilled chicken salad** Grilled chicken Spring mix Kale salad
2	Smoothie Multivitamin	**Grilled salmon lettuce wrap** Salmon Avocado salad	**Grilled salmon & green beans** Salmon Green beans
3	Smoothie Multivitamin	**Steak/chicken stir-fry** Steak or chicken Mixed vegetables (optional ½ cup quinoa)	**Steak/chicken & Broccoli** Grilled steak or chicken Broccoli
4	Smoothie Multivitamin	**Turkey Burger + Kale salad** Turkey burger Chunky kale salad ½ medium avocado	**Meatballs** Meatballs Mashed cauliflower green beans
5	Smoothie Multivitamin	**Grilled salmon & green beans** Salmon Green beans	**Grilled salmon wrap** Salmon Avocado salad Side salad
6	Smoothie Multivitamin	**Tabbouleh quinoa salad with hummus** Quinoa Hummus Whole wheat pita bread	**Quinoa & vegetable skewers** Quinoa Vegetable skewers Avocado salad
7	Smoothie Multivitamin	**Herb baked tofu with cauliflower** Tofu Mashed cauliflower Green beans	**Herb baked tofu with salad** Tofu Avocado salad Kale salad

Day 1

Upon Rising and before breakfast

- State affirmation, journal, and/or meditate for 15 minutes
- Detox drink follow by 1 cup of water or elixir
- 1 cup green tea or shot of wheat grass juice before exercise
- **Exercise**: 30 minutes cardio, based on fitness level
- Optional supplements with meals: multivitamin, 1000mg cod liver oil, 1000mg vitamin C, 1-2 caps pancreatic enzymes, and probiotics

Breakfast: Smoothie

- 20 oz. infused water

Lunch: Grilled rosemary chicken kabobs + cauliflower rice

- 4 oz. grilled chicken breast
- 3 cups grilled vegetables
- ½ cup cauliflower rice
- 20 oz. infused water

Dinner: Tossed Rosemary grilled chicken salad with avocado dressing

- 4 oz. grilled chicken breast
- 1 cup spring mix salad
- 1 cup chunky kale with cucumber, bell peppers, tomato
- Toss with 4 tbsp. avocado dressing
- 20 oz. infused water

1-2 hour(s) before or after dinner

- 15 min weight training
- Enema or colonic if necessary
- Hot bath with Epsom salts
- Detox drink + 10 oz. dandelion or detox tea

Day 2

Upon Rising and before breakfast

- State affirmation, journal, and/or meditate for 15 minutes
- Detox drink follow by 1 cup of water or elixir
- 1 cup green tea or shot of wheat grass juice before exercise
- **Exercise**: 30 minutes cardio, based on fitness level
- Optional supplements with meals: multivitamin, 1000mg cod liver oil, 1000mg vitamin C, 1-2 caps pancreatic enzymes and probiotics

Breakfast: Smoothie

- 20 oz. infused water

Lunch: Grilled salmon lettuce wrap with ½ cup avocado salad

- 3 oz. grilled wild caught salmon
- 1 large lettuce leaf, 1 slice tomato, 3 slices cucumber
- ½ cup avocado salad
- 20 oz. infused water

Dinner: Grilled salmon with sautéed green beans

- 4 oz. grilled wild caught salmon
- 2 cups sautéed green beans in 1 tbsp. olive oil
- 20 oz. infused water

1-2 hour(s) before or after dinner

- 10 min core & 10 min flexibility
- Enema or colonic if necessary
- Hot bath with Epsom salts
- Detox drink + 10 oz. dandelion or detox tea

Day 3
Upon Rising and before breakfast

- State affirmation, journal, and/or meditate for 15 minutes
- Detox drink follow by 1 cup of water or elixir
- 1 cup green tea or shot of wheat grass juice before exercise
- **Exercise**: 30 minutes cardio, based on fitness level
- Optional supplements with meals: multivitamin, 1000mg cod liver oil, 1000mg vitamin C, 1-2 caps pancreatic enzymes, and probiotics

Breakfast: Smoothie

- 20 oz. infused water

Lunch: Steak or chicken stir-fry + cauliflower rice

- 3 oz. chicken or steak
- 3 cups vegetables
- ½ cup cauliflower rice
- 20 oz. infused water

Dinner: Grilled chicken or steak with broccoli

- 4 oz. chicken or steak
- 2 cups steam broccoli (lightly steamed)
- 1 cup side salad with vinaigrette
- 20 oz. infused water

1-2 hour(s) before or after dinner

- 15 min weight training
- Enema or colonic if necessary
- Hot bath with Epsom salts
- Detox drink + 10 oz. dandelion or detox tea

Day 4

Upon Rising and before breakfast

- State affirmation, journal, and/or meditate for 15 minutes
- Detox drink follow by 1 cup of water or elixir
- 1 cup green tea or shot of wheat grass juice before exercise
- **Exercise**: 10,000 steps
- Optional supplements with meals: multivitamin, 1000mg cod liver oil, 1000mg vitamin C, 1-2 caps pancreatic enzymes, and probiotics

Breakfast: Smoothie

- 20 oz. infused water

Lunch: Turkey burger with chunky kale salad

- 3 oz. turkey burger (bunless)
- ½ medium avocado
- 2 cups chunky kale salad
- 20 oz. infused water

Dinner: Turkey meatballs with mashed cauliflower + side salad

- 4 oz. turkey meatballs
- ½ cup mashed cauliflower
- 1 cup spring mix salad
- 20 oz. infused water

1-2 hour(s) before or after dinner

- 10 min core & 10 min flexibility
- Enema or colonic if necessary
- Hot bath with Epsom salts
- Detox drink + 10 oz. dandelion or detox tea

Day 5
Upon Rising and before breakfast

- State affirmation, journal, and/or meditate for 15 minutes
- Detox drink follow by 1 cup of water or elixir
- 1 cup green tea or shot of wheat grass juice before exercise
- **Exercise**: 30 minutes cardio, based on fitness level
- Optional supplements with meals: multivitamin, 1000mg cod liver oil, 1000mg vitamin C, 1-2 caps pancreatic enzymes, and probiotics

Breakfast: Smoothie

- 20 oz. infused water

Lunch: Grilled salmon with green beans

- 3 oz. grilled salmon
- 2 cups sautéed green beans with ½ cup onions
- 1 cup side salad tossed with vinaigrette
- 20 oz. infused water

Dinner: Grilled salmon with large tossed salad

- 4 oz. grilled salmon
- Tossed salad: 1 cup romaine lettuce + 1 cup kale salad
- Tossed with vinaigrette
- 20 oz. infused water

1-2 hour(s) before or after dinner

- Squats
- Enema or colonic if necessary
- Hot bath with Epsom salts
- Detox drink + 10 oz. dandelion or detox tea

Day 6
Upon Rising and before breakfast
+ State affirmation, journal, and/or meditate for 15 minutes
+ Detox drink follow by 1 cup of water or elixir
+ 1 cup green tea or shot of wheat grass juice before exercise
+ **Exercise**: 30 minutes cardio, based on fitness level
+ Optional supplements with meals: multivitamin, 1000mg cod liver oil, 1000mg vitamin C, 1-2 caps pancreatic enzymes, and probiotics

Breakfast: Smoothie
+ 20 oz. infused water

Lunch: Tabbouleh quinoa salad with hummus
+ 1 cup tabbouleh quinoa
+ 4 tbsp. hummus
+ 1 toasted whole grain pita bread
+ 20 oz. infused water

Dinner: Quinoa & vegetable skewers
+ 1 cup cooked quinoa
+ 2-3 vegetable skewers (red pepper, red onions, mushrooms, zucchini)
+ 20 oz. infused water

1-2 hour(s) before or after dinner
+ 10 min core & 10 min flexibility
+ Enema or colonic if necessary
+ Hot bath with Epsom salts
+ Detox drink + 10 oz. dandelion or detox tea

Day 7
Upon Rising and before breakfast
- State affirmation, journal, and/or meditate for 15 minutes
- Detox drink follow by 1 cup of water or elixir
- 1 cup green tea or shot of wheat grass juice before exercise
- **Cardio**: Rest
- Optional supplements with meals: multivitamin, 1000mg cod liver oil, 1000mg vitamin C, 1-2 caps pancreatic enzymes, and probiotics

Breakfast: Smoothie
- 20 oz. infused water

Lunch: Herb baked tofu with mashed cauliflower + green beans
- 6 oz. baked tofu
- 1 cup mashed cauliflower
- 1 cup sautéed green beans
- 20 oz. infused water

Dinner: Herb baked tofu + avocado and green salad
- 6 oz. baked tofu
- 2 cups green salad
- ½ cup avocado salad
- 20 oz. infused water

1-2 hour(s) before or after dinner
- 10 minute Deep breathing
- Enema or colonic if necessary
- Hot bath with Epsom salts
- Detox drink + 10 oz. dandelion or detox tea

Week 2 – Cleansing Week

Day	Breakfast	Lunch	Dinner
8	Smoothie Multivitamin	**Pea soup + kale salad** Pea soup Chunky kale salad Avocado dressing	**Quinoa Salad** Sprouted quinoa Fennel grilled vegetables Side salad
9	Smoothie Multivitamin	**Veggie skewers + Cauliflower mashed** Veggie skewers Mashed cauliflower Dandelion salad	**Soup & salad** Veggie soup Kale & lettuce mix salad Tossed with vinaigrette
10	Smoothie Multivitamin	Lunch Smoothie	Dinner Smoothie (Try green garden smoothie)
11	Smoothie Multivitamin	Lunch Smoothie	Dinner Smoothie (Try green garden smoothie)
12	Smoothie Multivitamin	Lunch Smoothie	Dinner Smoothie (Try green garden smoothie)
13	Smoothie Multivitamin	**Pea soup + kale salad** Pea soup Chunky kale salad Avocado dressing	**Quinoa Salad** Sprouted quinoa Fennel grilled vegetables Side salad
14	Smoothie Multivitamin	**Veggie skewers + Cauliflower mashed** Veggie skewers Mashed cauliflower Dandelion salad	**Soup & salad** Veggie soup Kale & lettuce mix salad Tossed with vinaigrette

Drink alkaline or immune broths in between meals.

Week 3 – Reintroduction Week

Day	Breakfast	Lunch	Dinner
15	Smoothie Multivitamin	**Quinoa & vegetable skewers** Quinoa Vegetable skewers Avocado salad	**Herb baked tofu** Tofu Mashed cauliflower Side salad
16	Smoothie Multivitamin	**Grilled salmon wrap** Salmon Avocado salad Side salad	**Grilled salmon & green beans** Salmon Green beans
17	Smoothie Multivitamin	**Chicken kabobs + cauliflower rice** Chicken Mixed Vegetables Cauliflower	**Tossed grilled chicken salad** Grilled chicken Spring mix Kale salad
18	Smoothie Multivitamin	**Steak/chicken stir-fry** Steak or chicken Mixed vegetables (optional quinoa)	**Steak/chicken & Broccoli** Grilled steak or chicken Broccoli
19	Smoothie Multivitamin	**Turkey Burger + Kale salad** Turkey burger Chunky kale salad medium avocado	**Meatballs** Meatballs Mashed cauliflower green beans
20	Smoothie Multivitamin	**Grilled salmon wrap** Salmon Avocado (tomatoes, parsley, cucumber)	**Grilled salmon & green beans** Salmon Green beans
21	Smoothie Multivitamin	**Chicken kabobs + cauliflower rice** Chicken Mixed Vegetables Cauliflower	**Tossed grilled chicken salad** Grilled chicken Spring mix Kale salad

Day 15

Upon Rising and before breakfast

- State affirmation, journal, and/or meditate for 15 minutes
- Detox drink follow by 1 cup of water or elixir
- 1 cup green tea or shot of wheat grass juice before exercise
- **Exercise**: 30 minutes cardio, based on fitness level
- Optional supplements with meals: multivitamin, 1000mg cod liver oil, 1000mg vitamin C, 1-2 caps pancreatic enzymes, and probiotics

Breakfast: Smoothie

- 20 oz. infused water

Lunch: Quinoa & vegetable skewers

- 1 cup cooked quinoa
- 2-3 vegetable skewers
- ½ cup avocado salad
- 20 oz. infused water

Dinner: Herb baked tofu with mashed cauliflower + green beans

- 6 oz. baked tofu
- 1 cup mashed cauliflower
- 1 cup sautéed green beans
- 20 oz. infused water

1-2 hour(s) before or after dinner

- 15-20 min weight training
- Enema or colonic if necessary
- Hot bath with Epsom salts
- Detox drink + 10 oz. dandelion or detox tea

Day 16
Upon Rising and before breakfast

- State affirmation, journal, and/or meditate for 15 minutes
- Detox drink follow by 1 cup of water or elixir
- 1 cup green tea or shot of wheat grass juice before exercise
- **Exercise**: 30 minutes cardio, based on fitness level
- Optional supplements with meals: multivitamin, 1000mg cod liver oil, 1000mg vitamin C, 1-2 caps pancreatic enzymes and probiotics

Breakfast: Smoothie

- 20 oz. infused water

Lunch: Grilled salmon lettuce wrap with ½ cup avocado salad

- 3 oz. grilled wild caught salmon
- 1 large lettuce leaf, 1 slice tomato, 3 slices cucumber
- ½ cup avocado salad
- 20 oz. infused water

Dinner: Grilled salmon with sautéed green beans

- 4 oz. grilled wild caught salmon
- 2 cups sautéed green beans in 1 tbsp. olive oil
- 20 oz. infused water

1-2 hour(s) before or after dinner

- 10 min core & 10 min flexibility
- Enema or colonic if necessary
- Hot bath with Epsom salts
- Detox drink + 10 oz. dandelion or detox tea

Day 17
Upon Rising and before breakfast

- State affirmation, journal, and/or meditate for 15 minutes
- Detox drink follow by 1 cup of water or elixir
- 1 cup green tea or shot of wheat grass juice before exercise
- **Exercise**: 30 minutes cardio, based on fitness level
- Optional supplements with meals: multivitamin, 1000mg cod liver oil, 1000mg vitamin C, 1-2 caps pancreatic enzymes, and probiotics

Breakfast: Smoothie

- 20 oz. infused water

Lunch: Grilled Rosemary Chicken Kabobs + cauliflower rice

- 4 oz. chicken breast
- 3 cups grilled vegetables
- ½ cup cauliflower rice
- 20 oz. infused water

Dinner: Tossed Rosemary grilled chicken salad with avocado dressing

- 4 oz. grilled chicken breast
- 1 cup spring mix salad
- 1 cup chunky kale with cucumber, bell peppers, tomato
- Toss with 4 tbsp. avocado dressing
- 20 oz. infused water

1-2 hour(s) before or after dinner

- 15-20 min weight training
- Enema or colonic if necessary
- Hot bath with Epsom salts
- Detox drink + 10 oz. dandelion or detox tea

Day 18
Upon Rising and before breakfast
- State affirmation, journal, and/or meditate for 15 minutes
- Detox drink follow by 1 cup of water or elixir
- 1 cup green tea or shot of wheat grass juice before exercise
- **Exercise**: 10,000 steps
- Optional supplements with meals: multivitamin, 1000mg cod liver oil, 1000mg vitamin C, 1-2 caps pancreatic enzymes, and probiotics

Breakfast: Smoothie
- 20 oz. infused water

Lunch: Steak or chicken stir-fry + cauliflower rice
- 3 oz. chicken or steak
- 3 cups vegetables
- ½ cup cauliflower rice
- 20 oz. infused water

Dinner: Grilled chicken or steak with broccoli
- 4 oz. chicken or steak
- 2 cups steam broccoli (lightly steamed)
- 1 cup side salad with vinaigrette
- 20 oz. infused water

1-2 hour(s) before or after dinner
- 10 min core & 10 min flexibility
- Enema or colonic if necessary
- Hot bath with Epsom salts
- Detox drink + 10 oz. dandelion or detox tea

Day 19

Upon Rising and before breakfast

- State affirmation, journal, and/or meditate for 15 minutes
- Detox drink follow by 1 cup of water or elixir
- 1 cup green tea or shot of wheat grass juice before exercise
- **Exercise**: 30 minutes cardio, based on fitness level
- Optional supplements with meals: multivitamin, 1000mg cod liver oil, 1000mg vitamin C, 1-2 caps pancreatic enzymes, and probiotics

Breakfast: Smoothie

- 20 oz. infused water

Lunch: Turkey burger with chunky kale salad

- 3 oz. turkey burger (bunless)
- ½ medium avocado
- 2 cups chunky kale salad
- 20 oz. infused water

Dinner: Turkey meatballs with mashed cauliflower + side salad

- 4 oz. turkey meatballs
- ½ cup mashed cauliflower
- 1 cup spring mix salad
- 20 oz. infused water

1-2 hour(s) before or after dinner

- Lunges
- Enema or colonic if necessary
- Hot bath with Epsom salts
- Detox drink + 10 oz. dandelion or detox tea

Day 20
Upon Rising and before breakfast
- State affirmation, journal, and/or meditate for 15 minutes
- Detox drink follow by 1 cup of water or elixir
- 1 cup green tea or shot of wheat grass juice before exercise
- **Exercise**: 30 minutes cardio, based on fitness level
- Optional supplements with meals: multivitamin, 1000mg cod liver oil, 1000mg vitamin C, 1-2 caps pancreatic enzymes, and probiotics

Breakfast: Smoothie
- 20 oz. infused water

Lunch: Grilled salmon with green beans
- 3 oz. grilled salmon
- 2 cups sautéed green beans with ½ cup onions
- 1 cup side salad tossed with vinaigrette
- 20 oz. infused water

Dinner: Grilled salmon with large tossed salad
- 4 oz. grilled salmon
- Tossed salad: 1 cup romaine lettuce + 1 cup kale salad
- Tossed with vinaigrette
- 20 oz. infused water

1-2 hour(s) before or after dinner
- 10 min core & 10 min flexibility
- Enema or colonic if necessary
- Hot bath with Epsom salts
- Detox drink + 10 oz. dandelion or detox tea

Day 21

Upon Rising and before breakfast

- State affirmation, journal, and/or meditate for 15 minutes
- Detox drink follow by 1 cup of water or elixir
- 1 cup green tea or shot of wheat grass juice before exercise
- **Exercise**: 30 minutes cardio, based on fitness level
- Optional supplements with meals: multivitamin, 1000mg cod liver oil, 1000mg vitamin C, 1-2 caps pancreatic enzymes, and probiotics

Breakfast: Smoothie

- 20 oz. infused water

Lunch: Grilled Rosemary Chicken Kabobs + cauliflower rice

- 4 oz. chicken breast
- 3 cups grilled vegetables
- ½ cup cauliflower rice
- 20 oz. infused water

Dinner: Tossed Rosemary grilled chicken salad with avocado dressing

- 4 oz. grilled chicken breast
- 1 cup spring mix salad
- 1 cup chunky kale with cucumber, bell peppers, tomato
- Toss with 4 tbsp. avocado dressing
- 20 oz. infused water

1-2 hour(s) before or after dinner

- 10 minute Deep Breathing
- Enema or colonic if necessary
- Hot bath with Epsom salts
- Detox drink + 10 oz. dandelion or detox tea

Fat Burning Phase Brief Recap!

	Fat Burning Phase	*Challenges*
Diet & Nutrition	*No starches* *60/30/10-Fat/Protein/Carb* *4+ servings of healthy fats* *4-6 oz. protein* *60-70g carbs per day*	*No sugar Challenge* ♦ *No Chocolate* ♦ *No Cake* ♦ *No Sweeteners*
Exercise	*Cardio: Interval Training* *Strength: 20 minutes* *Core: 15 minutes* *Flexibility: 15 minutes*	*Squats challenge* *100 by day 21*
Mind/Body	*Affirmation / Meditation / Journal / Visualization / Self-work*	*Affirmation and visualization Challenge*

Reminder:

♦ No food after 7 pm or 3 hours before bed

♦ Keep carbs between 60 & 70 grams (g) per day.

♦ Concentrate on counting carbs (no starches allowed).

♦ All protein shakes should contain a maximum of 20g of carbs.

♦ You can substitute protein shake for healthy breakfast with 1-2 servings of essential fatty acids, 3-4 ounces of protein, and 20g of carbs.

♦ Check recipes in the Recipe section for daily meals.

Snacks

Snacks in between meals in the fat burning phase may accelerate metabolism and fat burning process. Your snacks are restricted to protein, fats, and low calorie carbs such as celery sticks, cherry tomatoes, leafy greens, bell peppers, etc.

- Do not snack on potato chips, sugary sweets, nutritionally depleted products, or foods high in carbs.
- Snack portions are not full meals; restrict calories to 200 or less.
- Carbs should not exceed 5-7g per snack.
- ***Count your carbs first then add protein and fat.***

Snack options:

- Protein shake (3g carbs total)
- High protein plate: (6g carbs): 2 slices nitrite free turkey bacon, 2 hard boil eggs, ¼ medium size avocado, 1 cup mushroom
- 2 hard boil eggs + 2 slices of cheese (6g carbs)
- 5-6 egg white scrambled with 1 cup spinach (3g carbs)
- 3-4 nitrite free turkey bacon + 1 cup sautéed kale (5g carbs)
- 1-2 Turkey sausages + 1 cup cherry tomatoes (6g carbs)
- 1-2 cup(s) side salad + protein tossed with vinaigrette (6g carbs)
- 2 Turkey slices wrap in cheese + olives (7g carbs)
- 1 Carrot or 1 celery stick with 1 oz. of cheese (4-7g carbs)

Week 4 Menu - Fat Burning Phase

Day	Breakfast	Lunch	Dinner
1	Protein Shake	**Rosemary chicken Stir fry** Chicken breast Mixed vegetables Cauliflower rice	**Tossed Rosemary chicken salad with vinaigrette** Chicken Breast Romaine & Kale Kalamata olives
2	Protein Shake	**Lemon grilled salmon lettuce wrap** Salmon Avocado salad	**Grilled salmon + green beans** Salmon Green beans
3	Protein Shake	**Bunless Turkey Burger + Kale salad** Ground turkey Avocado Kale chunky salad	**Zucchini stuffed ground turkey** Ground turkey Zucchini Goat cheese
4	Protein Shake	**Grilled Halibut + asparagus** Grilled Halibut Asparagus spears	**Grilled halibut spinach wrap** Grilled halibut Spinach Kale Avocado salad
5	Protein Shake	**Tossed Rosemary chicken salad with vinaigrette** Chicken Breast Romaine & Kale Kalamata olives	**Grilled Chicken & Veggie Skewers** Chicken Veggie Skewers Side salad
6	Protein Shake	**Lemon grilled salmon lettuce wrap** Salmon Avocado salad	**Grilled salmon + green beans** Salmon Green beans
7	Protein Shake	**Bunless Turkey Burger + Kale salad** Ground turkey Avocado Kale chunky salad	**Zucchini stuffed ground turkey** Ground turkey Zucchini Goat cheese

Day 1
Upon rising and before breakfast

- State affirmation, journal, and/or meditate
- Drink 10oz of warm infused water or apple cider vinegar elixir
- 1 cup green tea / black coffee or shot of wheat grass juice before exercise
- **Exercise**: 15 seconds **HIIT 1** (10, 15, or 20 rounds)

Breakfast: Protein Shake

- 1,000 mg fish oil or CLA
- Multivitamin
- 20 oz. infused water

Lunch: Rosemary Chicken Stir Fry + cauliflower rice

- 4 oz. chicken breast
- 3 cups vegetables (1 cup broccoli, ½ cup bell peppers, ½ cup onions, 1 cup asparagus)
- ½ cup cauliflower rice
- 20 oz. infused water

Dinner: Tossed Rosemary grilled chicken salad with avocado dressing

- 6 oz. grilled chicken breast
- 1 cup spring mix salad
- 1 cup chunky kale (½ cup cucumber, bell peppers, tomato)
- Toss with 4 tbsp. avocado dressing
- 20 oz. infused water

1-2 hour(s) before or after dinner

- 15 seconds **HIIT 4** core (10, 15, or 20 rounds)
- 15 min yoga / stretch
- 20 oz. infused water

Day 2
Upon rising and before breakfast
- State affirmation, journal, and/or meditate
- Drink 10oz infused water or apple cider vinegar elixir
- 1 cup green tea / black coffee or shot of wheat grass juice before exercise
- **Exercise**: Cardio interval training

Breakfast: Protein Shake
- 1,000 mg fish oil or CLA
- Multivitamin
- 20 oz. infused water

Lunch: Grilled lemon salmon lettuce wrap with avocado salad
- 2 (3 oz.) grilled lemon salmon wrap in 1-2 large loose leaf lettuce(s)
- ½ cup avocado salad (1 medium avocado, 1 tomato, 1 cucumber, ½ red onions, chopped parsley)
- 1 cup spring mix salad tossed with 1 tbsp. vinaigrette
- 20 oz. infused water

Dinner: Grilled lemon salmon with asparagus & mashed cauliflower
- 6 oz. grilled salmon
- 12 spears asparagus
- 1 cup mashed cauliflower (optional)
- 20 oz. infused water

1-2 hour(s) before or after dinner
- 25-minute upper body weight training
- 20 oz. infused water

Day 3
Upon rising and before breakfast

- State affirmation, journal, and/or meditate
- Drink 10oz infused water or apple cider vinegar elixir
- 1 cup green tea / black coffee or shot of wheat grass juice before exercise
- **Exercise**: 20 seconds each **HIIT 1** (10, 15, or 20 rounds)

Breakfast: Protein Shake

- 1,000 mg fish oil or CLA
- Multivitamin
- 20 oz. infused water

Lunch: Bunless Turkey Burger with kale salad

- 4 oz. turkey burger patty
- 2 slices of mozzarella cheese
- ½ medium avocado
- 1½ cups chunky kale (½ cup cucumber, bell peppers, tomato)
- 20 oz. infused water

Dinner: Ground Turkey stuffed Zucchini with side salad

- 6 oz. ground turkey
- 2 Zucchini
- 1 oz. goat cheese (sprinkle on top)
- 1 cup spring mix salad tossed with vinaigrette
- 20 oz. infused water

1-2 hour(s) before or after dinner

- 20 seconds **HIIT 4** core (10, 15, or 20 rounds)
- 15 min yoga / stretch
- 20 oz. infused water

Day 4
Upon rising and before breakfast
- State affirmation, journal, and/or meditate
- Drink 10oz infused water or apple cider vinegar elixir
- 1 cup green tea / black coffee or shot of wheat grass juice before exercise
- **Exercise**: Rest or 10,000 steps

Breakfast: Protein Shake
- 1,000 mg fish oil or CLA
- Multivitamin
- 20 oz. infused water

Lunch: Grilled halibut with asparagus
- 4 oz. grilled halibut
- 12 spears asparagus
- 1 cup cauliflower mashed
- 20 oz. infused water

Dinner: Grilled halibut sautéed spinach wrap
- 2 (3oz.) grilled halibut wrap in 2 large loose leaf lettuce(s)
- Sautéed spinach (2 cups spinach, ½ cup onions, ½ cup mushrooms) inside wrap
- 1 cup kale salad tossed with 1 tbsp. vinaigrette
- 20 oz. infused water

1-2 hour(s) before or after dinner
- 25 minute lower body weight training
- 20 oz. infused water

Day 5
Upon rising and before breakfast
- State affirmation, journal, and/or meditate
- Drink 10oz. infused water or apple cider vinegar elixir
- 1 cup green tea / black coffee or shot of wheat grass juice before exercise
- **Exercise**: 30 seconds **HIIT 1** (10, 15, or 20 rounds)

Breakfast: Protein Shake
- 1,000 mg fish oil or CLA
- Multivitamin
- 20 oz. infused water

Lunch: Rosemary Chicken Kabobs + cauliflower rice
- 1-2 skewer(s) - 4-5oz. chicken breast + vegetables
- Vegetables (1-2 cup(s) zucchini, bell peppers, red onions)
- 1 cup cauliflower rice
- 20 oz. infused water

Dinner: Tossed rosemary grilled chicken salad with avocado dressing
- 6 oz. grilled chicken breast
- 1 cup spring mix salad
- 1 cup chunky kale (½ cup cucumber, bell peppers, tomato)
- Toss with 4 tbsp. avocado dressing

1-2 hour(s) before or after dinner
- 30 seconds **HIIT 4** core (10, 15, or 20 rounds)
- 15 min yoga / stretch
- 20 oz. infused water

Day 6
Upon rising and before breakfast

- State affirmation, journal, and/or meditate
- Drink 10oz infused water or apple cider vinegar elixir
- 1 cup green tea / black coffee or shot of wheat grass juice before exercise
- **Exercise**: Cardio Interval Training

Breakfast: Protein Shake

- 1,000 mg fish oil or CLA
- 2 multivitamin
- 20 oz. infused water

Lunch: Grilled lemon salmon wrap with avocado salad

- 4 oz. grilled salmon wrap in 1-2 large loose leaf lettuce(s)
- Avocado salad (1 medium avocado, 1 tomato, 1 cucumber, ½ red onions, chopped parsley)
- 1 cup spring mix salad tossed with 1 tbsp. vinaigrette
- 20 oz. infused water

Dinner: Grilled lemon salmon with asparagus & cauliflower mashed

- 6 oz. grilled salmon
- 12 spears asparagus
- 1 cup cauliflower mashed
- 20 oz. infused water

1-2 hour(s) before or after dinner

- 25-minute upper body weight training
- 20 oz. infused water

Day 7
Upon rising and before breakfast
- State affirmation, journal, and/or meditate
- Drink 10oz infused water or apple cider vinegar elixir
- 1 cup green tea / black coffee or shot of wheat grass juice before exercise
- **Exercise**: 1 minute each **HIIT 1** (5, 10, or 15 rounds)

Breakfast: Protein Shake
- 1,000 mg fish oil or CLA
- Multivitamin
- 20 oz. infused water

Lunch: Bunless Turkey Burger with kale salad
- 4 oz. turkey burger patty
- 2 slices of mozzarella cheese
- ½ medium avocado
- 1½ cup chunky kale (½ cup cucumber, bell peppers, tomato)
- 20 oz. infused water

Dinner: Ground Turkey stuffed Zucchini with spring mix salad
- 6 oz. ground turkey
- 2 Zucchini
- 1 oz. goat cheese (sprinkle on top)
- 1 cup spring mix salad tossed with vinaigrette
- 20 oz. infused water

1-2 hour(s) before or after dinner
- 1 minute **HIIT 4** core (5, 10, or 15 rounds)
- 15 minute yoga/stretch
- 20 oz. infused water

Week 5 Menu – Fat Burning Phase

Day	Breakfast	Lunch	Dinner
8	Protein Shake Multivitamin 1000mg Fish/flax oil	**Dill Tuna Skewers** Tuna steak Sautéed spinach Onions and garlic Green salad	**Seared tuna + fennel salad** Tuna steak Fennel salad
9	Protein Shake Multivitamin 1000mg Fish/flax oil	**Tossed roasted chicken salad** Chicken Breast Romaine & Kale Goat cheese Kalamata olives	**Roasted chicken + asparagus** Chicken Breast Asparagus spears Spring mix lettuce
10	Protein Shake Multivitamin 1000mg Fish/flax oil	**Shrimp lettuce wrap** Shrimp Colorful slaw	**King prawns** (large Shrimp) King prawns Grilled Bok choy
11	Protein Shake Multivitamin 1000mg Fish/flax oil	**Portabella Buffalo Burger** Buffalo burger Portabella mushroom Broccoli	**Portabella Buffalo Burger** Buffalo burger Portabella mushroom Green salad
12	Protein Shake Multivitamin 1000mg Fish/flax oil	**Dill Tuna Skewers** Tuna steak Sautéed spinach Onions and garlic Green salad	**Seared tuna + fennel salad** Tuna steak Fennel salad
13	Protein Shake Multivitamin 1000mg Fish/flax oil	**Tossed roasted chicken salad with vinaigrette** Chicken Breast Romaine & Kale Goat cheese Kalamata olives	**Roasted chicken + asparagus** Chicken Breast Asparagus spears Spring mix lettuce
14	Protein Shake Multivitamin 1000mg Fish/flax oil	**Shrimp lettuce wrap** Shrimp Colorful slaw	**King prawns** (large Shrimp) King prawns Grilled Bok choy

Day 8
Upon rising and before breakfast

- State affirmation, journal, and/or meditate
- Drink 10oz infused water or apple cider vinegar elixir
- 1 cup green tea / black coffee or shot of wheat grass juice before exercise
- **Exercise**: 15 seconds **HIIT 2** (10, 15, or 20 rounds)

Breakfast: Protein Shake

- 1,000 mg fish oil or CLA
- Multivitamin
- 20 oz. infused water

Lunch: Dill Tuna Skewers with spinach + side salad

- 4 oz. tuna steak
- 2 cups sautéed spinach with olive oil and ½ cup onions
- 1 cup side salad
- 20 oz. infused water

Dinner: Seared tuna with shaved fennel salad

- 6 oz. seared tuna
- 2 cups fennel salad
- 20 oz. infused water

1-2 hour(s) before or after dinner

- 15 seconds **HIIT 4** (10, 15, or 20 rounds)
- 15 minute yoga/stretch

Day 9
Upon rising and before breakfast

- State affirmation, journal, and/or meditate
- Drink 10oz infused water or apple cider vinegar elixir
- 1 cup green tea / black coffee or shot of wheat grass juice before exercise
- **Exercise**: Cardio Interval Training

Breakfast: Protein Shake (20g carbs)

- 1,000 mg fish oil or CLA
- Multivitamin
- 20 oz. infused water

Lunch: Tossed roasted chicken salad goat cheese and avocado

- 4 oz. chicken breast
- Salad: (1 cup each spring mix salad, chopped broccoli, chopped purple cauliflower)
- 1 oz. goat cheese
- ½ medium avocado
- Tossed with apple cider vinaigrette
- 20 oz. infused water

Dinner: Roasted chicken with asparagus

- 6 oz. grilled chicken
- 12 spears asparagus
- 1 cup purple cauliflower mashed
- 20 oz. infused water

1-2 hour(s) before or after dinner

- 25 minute weight training
- 20 oz. infused water

Day 10
Upon rising and before breakfast

- State affirmation, journal, and/or meditate
- Drink 10oz infused water or apple cider vinegar elixir
- 1 cup green tea / black coffee or shot of wheat grass juice before exercise
- **Exercise**: 20 seconds **HIIT 2** (10, 15, or 20 rounds)

Breakfast: Protein Shake (20g carbs)

- 1,000 mg fish oil or CLA
- Multivitamin
- 20 oz. infused water

Lunch: Grilled shrimp lettuce wrap with colorful slaw

- 2 shrimp wraps
- ¼ cup colorful slaw
- ½ medium avocado
- 20 oz. infused water

Dinner: King prawns with grilled Bok choy

- 4 King prawns
- 2 whole Bok choy grilled with olive oil
- 1 cup side salad
- 20 oz. infused water

1-2 hour(s) before or after dinner

- 20 seconds **HIIT 4** core (10, 15, or 20 rounds)
- 15 minute yoga/stretch
- 20 oz. infused water

Day 11

Upon rising and before breakfast

- State affirmation, journal, and/or meditate
- Drink 10oz infused water or apple cider vinegar elixir
- 1 cup green tea / black coffee or shot of wheat grass juice before exercise
- **Exercise**: Rest or 10,000 steps

Breakfast: Protein Shake (20g carbs)

- 1,000 mg fish oil or CLA
- Multivitamin

Lunch: Portabella buffalo burger

- 4 oz. ground buffalo with blue cheese
- 2 cups steamed broccoli
- 20 oz. infused water

Dinner: Portabella buffalo burger

- 4 oz. ground buffalo with blue cheese
- 2 cups green salad
- 3 tbsp. avocado dressing

1-2 hour(s) before or after dinner

- 25 minute weight training
- 20 oz. infused water

Day 12

Upon rising and before breakfast

- State affirmation, journal, and/or meditate
- Drink 10oz infused water or apple cider vinegar elixir
- 1 cup green tea / black coffee or shot of wheat grass juice before exercise
- **Exercise**: 30 seconds **HIIT 2** (10, 15, or 20 rounds)

Breakfast: Protein Shake (20g carbs)

- 1,000 mg fish oil or CLA
- Multivitamin
- 20 oz. infused water

Lunch: Dill Tuna Skewers with spinach + side salad

- 4 oz. tuna steak
- 2 cups sautéed spinach with olive oil and ½ cup onions
- 1 cup side salad
- 20 oz. infused water

Dinner: Seared tuna with shaved fennel salad

- 6 oz. seared tuna
- 2 cups fennel salad
- 20 oz. infused water

1-2 hour(s) before or after dinner

- 30 seconds **HIIT 4** (10, 15, or 20 rounds)
- 15 minute yoga/stretch

Day 13
Upon rising and before breakfast

- State affirmation, journal, and/or meditate
- Drink 10oz infused water or apple cider vinegar elixir
- 1 cup green tea / black coffee or shot of wheat grass juice before exercise
- **Exercise**: Cardio Interval Training

Breakfast: Protein Shake (20g carbs)

- 1,000 mg fish oil or CLA
- Multivitamin
- 20 oz. infused water

Lunch: Tossed roasted chicken salad goat cheese and avocado

- 4 oz. chicken breast
- Salad: (1 cup each spring mix salad, chopped broccoli, chopped purple cauliflower)
- 1 oz. goat cheese
- ½ medium avocado
- Tossed with apple cider vinaigrette
- 20 oz. infused water

Dinner: Roasted chicken with asparagus

- 6 oz. grilled chicken
- 12 spears asparagus
- 1 cup purple cauliflower mashed
- 20 oz. infused water

1-2 hour(s) before or after dinner

- 25 minute weight training
- 20 oz. infused water

Day 14
Upon rising and before breakfast
- State affirmation, journal, and/or meditate
- Drink 10oz infused water or apple cider vinegar elixir
- 1 cup green tea / black coffee or shot of wheat grass juice before exercise
- **Exercise**: 1 minute **HIIT 2** (5, 10, or 15 rounds)

Breakfast: Protein Shake
- 1,000 mg fish oil or CLA
- Multivitamin
- 20 oz. infused water

Lunch: Grilled shrimp lettuce wrap with colorful slaw
- 2 shrimp wraps
- ¼ cup colorful slaw
- ½ medium avocado
- 20 oz. infused water

Dinner: King prawns with grilled Bok choy
- 4 King prawns
- 2 whole Bok choy grilled with olive oil
- 1 cup side salad
- 20 oz. infused water

1-2 hour(s) before or after dinner
- 1 minute **HIIT 4** core (5, 10, or 15rounds)
- 15 minute yoga/stretch
- 20 oz. infused water

Week 6 Menu - Fat Burning Phase

Day	Breakfast	Lunch	Dinner
15	Protein Shake Multivitamin 1000mg Fish/flax oil	**Scallops + avocado salad** Scallops Avocado salad	**Scallops + fennel salad** Scallops Fennel salad
16	Protein Shake Multivitamin 1000mg Fish/flax oil	**Dill Turkey Breast + veggies** Turkey breast grilled vegetables	**Dill Turkey Breast salad** Turkey breast Spinach Kale Vinaigrette
17	Protein Shake Multivitamin 1000mg Fish/flax oil	**Baked fish wrap + slaw** Fish (wrap in lettuce) Colorful slaw Medium avocado	**Baked Fish + asparagus** Fish Asparagus spears Side salad
18	Protein Shake Multivitamin 1000mg Fish/flax oil	**Lamb Kabobs** Lamb Grilled vegetables	**Lamb Kabobs** Lamb Spring mix Vinaigrette
19	Protein Shake Multivitamin 1000mg Fish/flax oil	**Scallops + avocado salad** Scallops Avocado salad	**Scallops + fennel salad** Scallops Fennel salad
20	Protein Shake Multivitamin 1000mg Fish/flax oil	**Dill Turkey Breast + veggies** Turkey breast grilled vegetables	**Dill Turkey Breast salad** Turkey breast Spinach Kale Vinaigrette
21	Protein Shake Multivitamin 1000mg Fish/flax oil	**Baked fish wrap + slaw** Fish (wrap in lettuce) Colorful slaw Medium avocado	**Baked Fish + asparagus** Fish Asparagus spears Side salad

Day 15
Upon rising and before breakfast
- State affirmation, journal, and/or meditate
- Drink 10oz infused water or apple cider vinegar elixir
- 1 cup green tea / black coffee or shot of wheat grass juice before exercise
- **Exercise**: 15 seconds **HIIT 3** (10, 15, or 20 rounds)

Breakfast: Protein Shake
- 1,000 mg fish oil or CLA
- Multivitamin
- 20 oz. infused water

Lunch: Scallops with avocado & side salad
- 4 oz. tuna steak
- ¼ cup avocado salad
- 1 cup side salad
- 20 oz. infused water

Dinner: Scallops with shaved fennel salad
- 6 oz. seared scallops
- 2 cups fennel salad
- 20 oz. infused water

1-2 hour(s) before or after dinner
- 15 seconds **HIIT 4** (10, 15, or 20 rounds)
- 15 minute yoga/stretch

Day 16
Upon rising and before breakfast

- State affirmation, journal, and/or meditate
- Drink 10oz infused water or apple cider vinegar elixir
- 1 cup green tea / black coffee or shot of wheat grass juice before exercise
- **Exercise**: Cardio Interval Training

Breakfast: Protein Shake

- 1,000 mg fish oil or CLA
- Multivitamin
- 20 oz. infused water

Lunch: Dill turkey breast with grilled vegetables

- 4 oz. turkey breast
- 2 cups grilled vegetables
- 1 cup side salad
- 20 oz. infused water

Dinner: Dill turkey breast salad

- 6 oz. grilled chicken
- 1 cup spinach
- 1 cup kale
- Toss in 2 tbsp. vinaigrette
- 20 oz. infused water

1-2 hour(s) before or after dinner

- 25 minute weight training
- 20 oz. infused water

Day 17
Upon rising and before breakfast
- State affirmation, journal, and/or meditate
- Drink 10oz infused water or apple cider vinegar elixir
- 1 cup green tea / black coffee or shot of wheat grass juice before exercise
- **Exercise**: 20 seconds **HIIT 3** (10, 15, or 20 rounds)

Breakfast: Protein Shake
- 1,000 mg fish oil or CLA
- Multivitamin
- 20 oz. infused water

Lunch: Bake fish lettuce wrap with colorful slaw
- 2 (3oz.) fish wraps
- 1 cup colorful slaw
- ½ medium avocado
- 20 oz. infused water

Dinner: Bake fish with grilled asparagus
- 6 oz. bake fish
- 12 lightly grilled asparagus spears
- 1 cup side salad
- 20 oz. infused water

1-2 hour(s) before or after dinner
- 20 seconds **HIIT 4** core (10, 15, or 20 rounds)
- 15 minute yoga/stretch
- 20 oz. infused water

Day 18
Upon rising and before breakfast

- State affirmation, journal, and/or meditate
- Drink 10oz infused water or apple cider vinegar elixir
- 1 cup green tea / black coffee or shot of wheat grass juice before exercise
- **Exercise**: Rest or 10,000 steps

Breakfast: Protein Shake

- 1,000 mg fish oil or CLA
- Multivitamin

Lunch: Lamb Kabobs with steamed broccoli

- 1-2 lamb kabobs
- 2 cups steamed broccoli
- 20 oz. infused water

Lunch: Lamb Kabobs with spring mix salad

- 2-3 lamb kabobs
- 2 cups spring mix salad
- 3 tbsp. avocado dressing

1-2 hour(s) before or after dinner

- 25 minute weight training
- 20 oz. infused water

Day 19
Upon rising and before breakfast

- State affirmation, journal, and/or meditate
- Drink 10oz infused water or apple cider vinegar elixir
- 1 cup green tea / black coffee or shot of wheat grass juice before exercise
- **Exercise**: 30 seconds **HIIT 3** (10, 15, or 20 rounds)

Breakfast: Protein Shake

- 1,000 mg fish oil or CLA
- Multivitamin
- 20 oz. infused water

Lunch: Scallops with avocado & side salad

- 4 oz. tuna steak
- ¼ cup avocado salad
- 1 cup side salad
- 20 oz. infused water

Dinner: Scallops with shaved fennel salad

- 6 oz. seared scallops
- 2 cups fennel salad
- 20 oz. infused water

1-2 hour(s) before or after dinner

- 30 seconds **HIIT 4** (10, 15, or 20 rounds)
- 15 minute yoga/stretch

Day 20
Upon rising and before breakfast
- State affirmation, journal, and/or meditate
- Drink 10oz infused water or apple cider vinegar elixir
- 1 cup green tea / black coffee or shot of wheat grass juice before exercise
- **Exercise**: Cardio Interval Training

Breakfast: Protein Shake
- 1,000 mg fish oil or CLA
- Multivitamin
- 20 oz. infused water

Lunch: Dill turkey breast with grilled vegetables
- 4 oz. turkey breast
- 2 cups grilled vegetables
- 1 cup side salad
- 20 oz. infused water

Dinner: Dill turkey breast salad
- 6 oz. grilled chicken
- 1 cup spinach
- 1 cup kale
- Toss in 2 tbsp. vinaigrette
- 20 oz. infused water

1-2 hour(s) before or after dinner
- 25 minute weight training
- 20 oz. infused water

Day 21
Upon rising and before breakfast
- State affirmation, journal, and/or meditate
- Drink 10oz infused water or apple cider vinegar elixir
- 1 cup green tea / black coffee or shot of wheat grass juice before exercise
- **Exercise**: 1 minute **HIIT 3** (5, 10, or 15 rounds)

Breakfast: Protein Shake
- 1,000 mg fish oil or CLA
- Multivitamin
- 20 oz. infused water

Lunch: Bake fish lettuce wrap with colorful slaw
- 2 (3oz.) fish wraps
- 1 cup colorful slaw
- ½ medium avocado
- 20 oz. infused water

Dinner: Bake fish with grilled asparagus
- 6 oz. bake fish
- 12 lightly grilled asparagus spears
- 1 cup side salad
- 20 oz. infused water

1-2 hour(s) before or after dinner
- 20 minute **HIIT 4** core (5, 10, or 15 rounds)
- 15 minute yoga/stretch
- 20 oz. infused water

Weight Mastery / Healthy 4 Life Phase Brief Recap!

	Weight Mastery Phase	*Challenges*
Diet & Nutrition	*Low starch* *Moderate protein* *2 vegetarian meals / week* *20/40/40 Fat/Protein/Carbs* *Total carb per day = 150g*	***Healthy 4 Life Challenge*** *Commitment to eating healthy daily*
Exercise	*Cardio: Alternating Interval Training & Regular Cardio* *Strength: 35 minutes* *Core: 20 minutes* *Flexibility: 20 minutes*	***The Big 100 Challenge*** *Start with 100 and add 100 per week*
Mind/Body	*Affirmation / Meditation / Journal / Visualization / Self-work*	***Pamper Yourself Challenge***

Reminder:

- No food after 7 pm or 3 hours before bed
- Concentrate healthy eating.
- Try adding vegetarian meals.
- You can substitute protein shake for healthy breakfast with 1-2 servings of essential fatty acids, 3-4 ounces of protein, and 20g of carbs.
- Check recipes in the Recipe section for daily meals.

Snacks

Healthy snacks in the weight mastery phase may continue to increase metabolism. Keep your snacks healthy and high in protein. Do not snack on foods high in carbs, potato chips, sugary sweets, or nutritionally depleted products. Remember snack portions are not full meals; restrict calories to about 200 or less.

Your snack options include:

- Chia seeds pudding parfait
- Celery sticks with almond butter
- 10-15 almonds with 3-4 strawberries
- Small side salad with protein
- Seaweed salad
- 1-2 cups of Soup
- 1 cup infused water or freshly made juice

Breakfast Options:

- 2-3 hard boil eggs with 2 slices of tomatoes
- 5 egg white scrambled with spinach
- 3-4 nitrite free turkey bacon with side steamed vegetables
- Scrambled tofu with vegetables
- Turkey sausage with sautéed vegetables
- Chia seeds pudding parfait
- Smoothie
- Protein shake
- Oatmeal with berries and walnuts

Week 7 Menu – Weight Mastery / Healthy 4 Life Phase

Day	Breakfast	Lunch	Dinner
1	Protein Shake	**Rosemary chicken Stir fry** Chicken breast Vegetables Brown rice	**Tossed Rosemary chicken salad** Chicken Breast Romaine & Kale Kalamata olives
2	Protein Shake	**Lemon grilled salmon lettuce wrap** Salmon Avocado salad Side salad	**Grilled salmon with asparagus & sweet potato** Salmon Asparagus Sweet potato
3	Protein Shake	**Bunless Turkey Burger + Kale salad** Ground turkey Medium avocado Chunky kale salad	**Zucchini stuffed ground turkey** Ground turkey Zucchini Side salad
4	Protein Shake	**Herb baked Sesame Tofu** Tofu Asparagus spears Brown rice	**Herb baked tofu** Tofu Grilled vegetables Side salad
5	Protein Shake	**Rosemary chicken Stir fry** Chicken breast Vegetables Brown rice	**Tossed Rosemary chicken salad with vinaigrette** Chicken Breast Romaine & Kale Kalamata olives
6	Protein Shake	**Lemon grilled salmon lettuce wrap** Salmon Avocado salad Side salad	**Grilled salmon with asparagus & sweet potato** Salmon Asparagus Sweet potato
7	Protein Shake	**Bunless Turkey Burger + Kale salad** Ground turkey Medium avocado Chunky kale salad	**Zucchini stuffed ground turkey** Ground turkey Zucchini Side salad

Day 1

Upon rising and before breakfast

- State affirmation, journal, and/or meditate
- Drink 10oz. of warm infused water or apple cider vinegar elixir
- 1 cup green tea / black coffee or shot of wheat grass juice before exercise
- **Exercise**: 30-45 minutes cardio

Breakfast: Protein Shake

- 1,000 mg fish oil or CLA
- Multivitamin
- 20 oz. infused water

Lunch: Rosemary Chicken Stir Fry with brown rice

- 4 oz. chicken breast
- 2 cups vegetables (1 cup broccoli, ½ cup bell peppers, ½ cup onions, 1 cup asparagus)
- 1 cup brown rice
- 20 oz. infused water

Dinner: Tossed Rosemary grilled chicken salad with avocado dressing (20g carbs)

- 4 oz. grilled chicken breast
- 1 cup spring mix salad
- 1 cup chunky kale (½ cup cucumber, bell peppers, tomato)
- Toss with 4 tbsp. avocado dressing
- 20 oz. infused water

1-2 hour(s) before or after dinner

- 35 minutes weight-training
- 20 oz. infused water

Day 2

Upon rising and before breakfast

- State affirmation, journal, and/or meditate
- Drink 10oz infused water or apple cider vinegar elixir
- 1 cup green tea / black coffee or shot of wheat grass juice before exercise
- **Exercise**: 20-30 minutes interval training

Breakfast: Protein Shake

- 1,000 mg fish oil or CLA
- Multivitamin
- 20 oz. infused water

Lunch: Grilled lemon salmon lettuce wrap with avocado salad

- 2 (3 oz.) grilled lemon salmon wrap in 1-2 large loose leaf lettuce(s)
- ½ cup avocado salad (1 medium avocado, 1 tomato, 1 cucumber, ½ red onions, chopped parsley)
- 1 cup spring mix salad tossed with 1 tbsp. vinaigrette
- 20 oz. infused water

Dinner: Grilled lemon salmon with baked sweet potato and asparagus

- 4 oz. grilled salmon
- 1 cup side salad
- 1 baked potato
- 20 oz. infused water

1-2 hour(s) before or after dinner

- 4-5 sets of 5 min abs, 20 minute flexibility training
- 20 oz. infused water

Day 3
Upon rising and before breakfast
♦ State affirmation, journal, and/or meditate
♦ Drink 10oz infused water or apple cider vinegar elixir
♦ 1 cup green tea / black coffee or shot of wheat grass juice before exercise
♦ **Exercise**: 30-45 minutes cardio

Breakfast: Protein Shake
♦ 1,000 mg fish oil or CLA
♦ Multivitamin
♦ 20 oz. infused water

Lunch: Bunless Turkey Burger with kale salad
♦ 4 oz. turkey burger patty
♦ 2 slices of mozzarella cheese
♦ ½ medium avocado
♦ 1½ cups chunky kale (½ cup cucumber, bell peppers, tomato)
♦ 20 oz. infused water

Dinner: Ground Turkey stuffed Zucchini with side salad
♦ 6 oz. ground turkey
♦ 2 Zucchini
♦ 1 oz. goat cheese (sprinkle on top)
♦ 1 cup spring mix salad tossed with vinaigrette
♦ 20 oz. infused water

1-2 hour(s) before or after dinner
♦ 35 minutes weight training
♦ 20 oz. infused water

Day 4
Upon rising and before breakfast

- State affirmation, journal, and/or meditate
- Drink 10oz infused water or apple cider vinegar elixir
- 1 cup green tea / black coffee or shot of wheat grass juice before exercise
- **Exercise**: 20-30 minutes interval training

Breakfast: Protein shake

- 20 oz. infused water

Lunch: Herb baked tofu with mashed cauliflower + green beans

- 6 oz. baked tofu
- 1 cup mashed cauliflower
- 1 cup sautéed green beans
- 20 oz. infused water

Dinner: Herb baked tofu + avocado and green salad

- 6 oz. baked tofu
- 2 cups green salad
- ½ cup avocado salad
- 20 oz. infused water

1-2 hour(s) before or after dinner

- 4-5 sets of 5 min abs, 20 minute flexibility training
- Enema or colonic if necessary
- Hot bath with Epsom salts
- 20 oz. infused water

Day 5
Upon rising and before breakfast

- State affirmation, journal, and/or meditate
- Drink 10oz. of warm infused water or apple cider vinegar elixir
- 1 cup green tea / black coffee or shot of wheat grass juice before exercise
- **Exercise**: 30-45 minutes cardio

Breakfast: Protein Shake

- 1,000 mg fish oil or CLA
- Multivitamin
- 20 oz. infused water

Lunch: Rosemary Chicken Stir Fry with brown rice

- 4 oz. chicken breast
- 2 cups vegetables (1 cup broccoli, ½ cup bell peppers, ½ cup onions, 1 cup asparagus)
- 1 cup brown rice
- 20 oz. infused water

Dinner: Tossed Rosemary grilled chicken salad with avocado dressing

- 4 oz. grilled chicken breast
- 1 cup spring mix salad
- 1 cup chunky kale (½ cup cucumber, bell peppers, tomato)
- Toss with 4 tbsp. avocado dressing
- 20 oz. infused water

1-2 hour(s) before or after dinner

- 35 minutes weight-training
- 20 oz. infused water

Day 6
Upon rising and before breakfast

- State affirmation, journal, and/or meditate
- Drink 10oz infused water or apple cider vinegar elixir
- 1 cup green tea / black coffee or shot of wheat grass juice before exercise
- **Exercise**: 20-30 minutes interval training

Breakfast: Protein Shake

- 1,000 mg fish oil or CLA
- Multivitamin
- 20 oz. infused water

Lunch: Grilled halibut lettuce wrap with avocado salad

- 2 (3 oz.) grilled halibut wrap in 1-2 large loose leaf lettuce(s)
- ½ cup avocado salad ((1 medium avocado, 1 tomato, 1 cucumber, ½ red onions, chopped parsley)
- 1 cup spring mix salad tossed with 1 tbsp. vinaigrette
- 20 oz. infused water

Dinner: Grilled halibut with baked sweet potato and asparagus

- 4 oz. grilled salmon
- 6 asparagus spears
- 1 baked potato
- 20 oz. infused water

1-2 hour(s) before or after dinner

- 4-5 sets of 5 min abs, 20 minute flexibility training
- 20 oz. infused water

Day 7
Upon rising and before breakfast

- State affirmation, journal, and/or meditate
- Drink 10oz infused water or apple cider vinegar elixir
- 1 cup green tea / black coffee or shot of wheat grass juice before exercise
- **Exercise**: 10,000 steps

Breakfast: Protein Shake

- 1,000 mg fish oil or CLA
- Multivitamin
- 20 oz. infused water

Lunch: Bunless Turkey Burger with kale salad

- 4 oz. turkey burger patty
- 2 slices of mozzarella cheese
- ½ medium avocado
- 1½ cups chunky kale (½ cup cucumber, bell peppers, tomato)
- 20 oz. infused water

Dinner: Ground Turkey stuffed Zucchini with side salad

- 6 oz. ground turkey
- 2 Zucchini
- 1 oz. goat cheese (sprinkle on top)
- 1 cup spring mix salad tossed with vinaigrette
- 20 oz. infused water

1-2 hour(s) before or after dinner

- Deep Breathing
- 20 oz. infused water

Week 8 menu - Weight Mastery / Healthy 4 Life Phase

Day	Breakfast	Lunch	Dinner
8	Protein Shake	**Dill Tuna Skewers** Tuna steak Grilled zucchini & squash	**Seared tuna + fennel salad** Tuna steak Fennel salad
9	Protein Shake	**Tossed roasted chicken & vegetable salad** Chicken Breast Broccoli & peppers Chunky kale salad	**Roasted chicken + asparagus** Chicken Green beans Mix green salad
10	Protein Shake	**Veggie skewers with quinoa** Veggie skewers Quinoa Side salad with walnuts	**Portabella Buffalo Burger** Buffalo burger Portabella mushrooms Slice cheese Side salad
11	Protein Shake	**Portabella Buffalo Burger** Buffalo burger Portabella mushrooms Bake sweet potato	**Veggie skewers with quinoa** Veggie skewers Quinoa Side salad with walnuts
12	Protein Shake	**Dill Tuna Skewers** Tuna steak Grilled zucchini & squash	**Seared tuna + fennel salad** Tuna steak Fennel salad
13	Protein Shake	**Tossed roasted chicken & vegetable salad** Chicken Breast Broccoli & peppers Chunky kale salad	**Roasted chicken + asparagus** Chicken Green beans Mix green salad
14	Protein Shake	**Shrimp Stir fry** Shrimp Vegetables Quinoa	**King prawns with sautéed spinach** King prawns Sautéed spinach with onions and garlic

Day 8
Upon rising and before breakfast

- State affirmation, journal, and/or meditate
- Drink 10oz infused water or apple cider vinegar elixir
- 1 cup green tea / black coffee or shot of wheat grass juice before exercise
- **Exercise**: Cardio 45 minutes

Breakfast: Protein Shake (20g carbs)

- 1,000 mg fish oil or CLA
- Multivitamin
- 20 oz. infused water

Lunch: Dill Tuna Skewers with spinach + side salad

- 4 oz. tuna steak
- 2 cups grilled zucchini and yellow squash
- 1 cup side salad with vinaigrette
- 20 oz. infused water

Dinner: Seared tuna with shaved fennel salad

- 4 oz. seared tuna
- 2 cups fennel salad
- 20 oz. infused water

1-2 hour(s) before or after dinner

- 35 minutes weight training
- 20 oz. water

Day 9
Upon rising and before breakfast

- State affirmation, journal, and/or meditate
- Drink 10 oz. infused water or apple cider vinegar elixir
- 1 cup green tea / black coffee or shot of wheat grass juice before exercise
- **Exercise**: Interval Training

Breakfast: Protein Shake

- 1,000 mg fish oil or CLA
- Multivitamin
- 20 oz. infused water

Lunch: Tossed roasted chicken and vegetable salad

- 4 oz. chicken breast
- 2 cups roasted broccoli and peppers
- 1 cup chunky kale
- ½ medium avocado
- Toss with apple cider vinaigrette
- 20 oz. infused water

Dinner: Roasted chicken with green beans

- 6 oz. grilled chicken
- 2 cups green beans
- 1 cup mix green salad
- 20 oz. infused water

1-2 hour(s) before or after dinner

- 4-5 sets 5 min abs
- 20 minute yoga
- 20 oz. infused water

Day 10
Upon rising and before breakfast

- State affirmation, journal, and/or meditate
- Drink 10 oz. infused water or apple cider vinegar elixir
- 1 cup green tea / black coffee or shot of wheat grass juice before exercise
- **Exercise**: 45 minutes cardio

Breakfast: Protein Shake

- 1,000 mg fish oil or CLA
- Multivitamin
- 20 oz. infused water

Lunch: Veggie skewers with quinoa

- 2-3 veggie skewers
- 1 cup quinoa
- 1 cup side salad
- 20 oz. infused water

Dinner: Portabella buffalo burger

- 4 oz. buffalo burger
- 2 portabella mushrooms
- 1 slice mozzarella cheese
- 1 cup side salad
- 20 oz. infused water

1-2 hour(s) before or after dinner

- 35 minutes weight training
- 20 oz. infused water

Day 11

Upon rising and before breakfast

- State affirmation, journal, and/or meditate
- Drink 10oz infused water or apple cider vinegar elixir
- 1 cup green tea / black coffee or shot of wheat grass juice before exercise
- **Exercise**: Rest or 10,000 steps

Breakfast: Protein Shake (20g carbs)

- 1,000 mg fish oil or CLA
- Multivitamin

Lunch: Portabella buffalo burger

- 4 oz. ground buffalo with blue cheese
- 2 portabella mushrooms
- 1 slice mozzarella cheese
- 1 Bake sweet potatoes
- 1 cup side salad
- 20 oz. infused water

Dinner: Veggie skewers with quinoa

- 2-3 veggie skewers
- 1 cup quinoa
- 1 cup side salad
- 20 oz. infused water

1-2 hour(s) before or after dinner

- 4-5 sets 5 min abs
- 20 minute yoga
- 20 oz. infused water

Day 12
Upon rising and before breakfast
- State affirmation, journal, and/or meditate
- Drink 10oz infused water or apple cider vinegar elixir
- 1 cup green tea / black coffee or shot of wheat grass juice before exercise
- **Exercise**: Cardio 45 minutes

Breakfast: Protein Shake (20g carbs)
- 1,000 mg fish oil or CLA
- Multivitamin
- 20 oz. infused water

Lunch: Dill Tuna Skewers with spinach + side salad
- 4 oz. tuna steak
- 2 cups grilled zucchini and squash
- 20 oz. infused water

Dinner: Seared tuna with shaved fennel salad
- 4 oz. seared tuna
- 2 cups fennel salad
- 20 oz. infused water

1-2 hour(s) before or after dinner
- 35 minutes weight training
- 20 oz. infused water

Day 13
Upon rising and before breakfast
- State affirmation, journal, and/or meditate
- Drink 10 oz. infused water or apple cider vinegar elixir
- 1 cup green tea / black coffee or shot of wheat grass juice before exercise
- **Exercise**: Interval Training

Breakfast: Protein Shake
- 1,000 mg fish oil or CLA
- Multivitamin
- 20 oz. infused water

Lunch: Tossed roasted chicken and vegetable salad
- 4 oz. chicken breast
- 1 cup roasted broccoli and peppers
- 1 cup chunky kale
- ½ medium avocado
- Toss with apple cider vinaigrette
- 20 oz. infused water

Dinner: Roasted chicken with green beans
- 6 oz. grilled chicken
- 2 cups green beans
- 1 cup mix green salad
- 20 oz. infused water

1-2 hour(s) before or after dinner
- 4-5 sets 5 min abs
- 20 minute stretch
- 20 oz. infused water

Day 14

Upon rising and before breakfast

- ♦ State affirmation, journal, and/or meditate
- ♦ Drink 10oz infused water or apple cider vinegar elixir
- ♦ 1 cup green tea / black coffee or shot of wheat grass juice before exercise
- ♦ **Exercise**: 10,000 steps

Breakfast: Protein Shake (20g carbs)

- ♦ 1,000 mg fish oil or CLA
- ♦ Multivitamin
- ♦ 20 oz. infused water

Lunch: Shrimp stir-fry with side quinoa

- ♦ 4 oz. shrimp
- ♦ 3 cups vegetables
- ♦ ½ cup quinoa or brown rice
- ♦ 20 oz. infused water

Dinner: King prawns with grilled Bok choy

- ♦ 4 King prawns
- ♦ 2 whole Bok choy grilled with olive oil
- ♦ 1 cup side salad
- ♦ 20 oz. infused water

1-2 hour(s) before or after dinner

- ♦ Deep Breathing
- ♦ 20 oz. infused water

Week 9 Menu – Weight Mastery / Healthy 4 Life Phase

Day	Breakfast	Lunch	Dinner
15	Smoothie Multivitamin	**Spaghetti squash with vegetables** Spaghetti squash 2-3 vegetable skewers	**3 bean taco salad** Black, pinto, red Lettuce & tomatoes Avocado salad
16	Smoothie Multivitamin	**Grilled salmon wrap** Salmon Medium avocado Side salad	**Grilled salmon & green beans** Salmon Green beans
17	Smoothie Multivitamin	**Chicken kabobs with brown rice** Chicken Breast Vegetables Brown rice	**Tossed grilled chicken salad** Grilled chicken breast Spring mix Kale salad Avocado dressing
18	Smoothie Multivitamin	**Steak stir-fry** Steak or chicken Vegetables	**Steak & peppers with broccoli** Grilled steak Broccoli Side salad
19	Smoothie Multivitamin	**Turkey Burger + Kale salad** Turkey burger Chunky kale salad Medium avocado	**Meatballs** Meatballs Green beans Bake sweet potato
20	Smoothie Multivitamin	**Grilled salmon wrap** Salmon Medium avocado Side salad	**Grilled salmon & green beans** Salmon Green beans
21	Smoothie Multivitamin	**Chicken kabobs with brown rice** Chicken Breast Vegetables Brown rice	**Tossed grilled chicken salad** Grilled chicken breast Spring mix Kale salad Avocado dressing

Day 15
Upon Rising and before breakfast
- State affirmation, journal, and/or meditate
- Drink 10 oz. warm infused water or apple cider vinegar elixir
- 1 cup green tea / black coffee or shot of wheat grass juice before exercise
- **Exercise**: 45 minutes cardio

Breakfast: Protein shake
- 1,000 mg fish oil or CLA
- Multivitamin
- 20 oz. infused water

Lunch: Spaghetti squash & vegetable skewers
- Bake spaghetti squash with olive oil
- 2-3 vegetable skewers
- Sprinkle flax seed meal
- (optional pasta sauce)
- 20 oz. infused water

Dinner: Herb baked tofu with mashed cauliflower + green beans
- 6 oz. baked tofu
- 1 cup mashed cauliflower
- 1 cup sautéed green beans
- 20 oz. infused water

1-2 hour(s) before or after dinner
- 35 minutes weight training
- 20 oz. infused water

Day 16

Upon rising and before breakfast

- State affirmation, journal, and/or meditate
- Drink 10 oz. warm infused water or apple cider vinegar elixir
- 1 cup green tea / black coffee or shot of wheat grass juice before exercise
- **Exercise**: 20-30 minutes interval training

Breakfast: Protein shake

- 1,000 mg fish oil or CLA
- Multivitamin
- 20 oz. infused water

Lunch: Grilled salmon lettuce wrap with avocado and side salad

- 3 oz. grilled wild caught salmon
- 1 large lettuce leaf, 1 slice tomato, 3 slices cucumber
- ½ medium avocado
- 1 cup side salad
- 20 oz. infused water

Dinner: Grilled salmon with sautéed green beans

- 4 oz. grilled wild caught salmon
- 2 cups sautéed green beans in 1 tbsp. olive oil
- 20 oz. infused water

1-2 hour(s) before or after dinner

- 4-5 sets 5 min abs
- 20 minute yoga
- 20 oz. infused water

Day 17
Upon rising and before breakfast
- State affirmation, journal, and/or meditate
- Drink 10 oz. warm infused water or apple cider vinegar elixir
- 1 cup green tea / black coffee or shot of wheat grass juice before exercise
- **Exercise**: 45 minutes cardio

Breakfast: Protein shake
- 1,000 mg fish oil or CLA
- Multivitamin
- 20 oz. infused water

Lunch: Grilled rosemary chicken kabobs with a side of brown rice
- 4 oz. chicken breast
- 2 cups grilled vegetables (1 cup broccoli, ½ cup bell peppers, ½ cup onions, 1 cup asparagus)
- ½ cup brown rice
- 20 oz. infused water

Dinner: Tossed rosemary grilled chicken salad with avocado dressing
- 4 oz. grilled chicken breast
- 1 cup spring mix salad
- 1 cup chunky kale with cucumber, bell peppers, tomato
- Toss with 4 tbsp. avocado dressing
- 20 oz. infused water

1-2 hour(s) before or after dinner
- 35 minutes weight training
- 20 oz. infused water

Day 18

Upon rising and before breakfast

- State affirmation, journal, and/or meditate
- Drink 10 oz. warm infused water or apple cider vinegar elixir
- 1 cup green tea / black coffee or shot of wheat grass juice before exercise
- **Exercise**: 20-30 minutes interval training

Breakfast: Protein shake

- 1,000 mg fish oil or CLA
- Multivitamin
- 20 oz. infused water

Lunch: Steak stir-fry

- 3 oz. chicken or steak
- 3 cups vegetables
- 20 oz. infused water

Dinner: Grilled steak and peppers with broccoli

- 4 oz. grilled steak
- 1 cup grilled red peppers
- 2 cups steam broccoli (lightly steamed)
- 1 cup side salad with vinaigrette
- 20 oz. infused water

1-2 hour(s) before or after dinner

- 4-5 sets 5 min abs
- 20 minute yoga
- 20 oz. infused water

Day 19

Upon Rising and before breakfast

- State affirmation, journal, and/or meditate
- Drink 10 oz. warm infused water or apple cider vinegar elixir
- 1 cup green tea / black coffee or shot of wheat grass juice before exercise
- **Exercise**: 45 minutes cardio

Breakfast: Protein shake

- 1,000 mg fish oil or CLA
- Multivitamin
- 20 oz. infused water

Lunch: Turkey burger with chunky kale salad

- 3 oz. turkey burger (bunless)
- ½ medium avocado
- 2 cups chunky kale salad
- 20 oz. infused water

Dinner: Turkey meatballs with sweet potato mashed + side salad

- 4 oz. turkey meatballs
- 1 baked sweet potato mashed
- 1 cup spring mix salad
- 20 oz. infused water

1-2 hour(s) before or after dinner

- 35 minutes weight training
- 20 oz. infused water

Day 20

Upon rising and before breakfast

- State affirmation, journal, and/or meditate
- Drink 10 oz. warm infused water or apple cider vinegar elixir
- 1 cup green tea / black coffee or shot of wheat grass juice before exercise
- **Exercise**: 20-30 minutes interval training

Breakfast: Protein shake

- 1,000 mg fish oil or CLA
- Multivitamin
- 20 oz. infused water

Lunch: Grilled salmon lettuce wrap with avocado & side salad

- 3 oz. grilled wild caught salmon
- 1 large lettuce leaf, 1 slice tomato, 3 slices cucumber
- ½ medium avocado
- 1 cup side salad
- 20 oz. infused water

Dinner: Grilled salmon with sautéed green beans

- 4 oz. grilled wild caught salmon
- 2 cups sautéed green beans in 1 tbsp. olive oil
- 20 oz. infused water

1-2 hour(s) before or after dinner

- 4-5 sets 5 min abs
- 20 minute yoga
- 20 oz. infused water

Day 21
Upon rising and before breakfast

- State affirmation, journal, and/or meditate
- Drink 10 oz. warm infused water or apple cider vinegar elixir
- 1 cup green tea / black coffee or shot of wheat grass juice before exercise
- **10,000 steps**

Breakfast: Protein shake

- 1,000 mg fish oil or CLA
- Multivitamin
- 20 oz. infused water

Lunch: Grilled rosemary chicken kabobs with a side of brown rice

- 4 oz. chicken breast
- 2 cups grilled vegetables (1 cup broccoli, ½ cup bell peppers, ½ cup onions, 1 cup asparagus)
- ½ cup brown rice
- 20 oz. infused water

Dinner: Tossed rosemary grilled chicken salad with avocado dressing

- 4 oz. grilled chicken breast
- 1 cup spring mix salad
- 1 cup chunky kale with cucumber, bell peppers, tomato
- Toss with 4 tbsp. avocado dressing
- 20 oz. infused water

1-2 hour(s) before or after dinner

- Deep breathing
- 20 oz. infused water

Recipes

❀ ❀ ❀

Morning Elixir (drink)

Choose from the following:

- ◆ 8oz warm water + ½ lemon + 1apple cider vinegar + 1/8 tsp/pinch cayenne pepper
- ◆ Chamomile tea
- ◆ Dandelion tea
- ◆ Freshly squeezed fruit juice or vegetable juice
- ◆ Warm water with lemon
- ◆ Infused water

Infused water recipes

Add any one or multiple of these simple recipes to 1 gallon of water and enjoy throughout the day.

2 whole lemon or lime, sliced

1 whole orange, sliced

2 lemon or lime with peppermint leaves

1 cucumber, sliced

4 strawberries, sliced

Lemon wedges, peppermint leaves, and ginger, sliced

A few slices of water melon

Detox Drink

2 ounces of unfiltered organic apple juice

2 ounces of aloe vera juice

4 ounces of warm pure / distilled water

1 tbsp. of bentonite clay

1 tsp psyllium husk or slippery elm

Use a blender bottle, pour in apple juice, aloe vera juice, and water. Add bentonite clay and psyllium husk to liquid mixture then shake well. Drink quickly as fiber will expand forming goo. Drink once in the morning and once at night.

Immediately after: Drink 10 ounces of pure water + 1 tbsp. lemon juice

Alkaline broth

3 celery stalks
2 cups spinach
2 cups kale
2 cups broccoli
1 bunch parsley
2 quarts water
Sea salt to taste

Place all vegetables in a large stockpot cover with cold water. Cook at low heat for 45minutes-1 hour. Add salt and let cook for another 10 minutes. Strain and keep the broth. This will keep in the refrigerator for 3 days. **Do not freeze and defrost**. Make fresh as needed.

Immune Booster Broth

½ pound mushrooms (variety – shiitake, oyster, cremini, portabella, bottom; at least 4)
2 large carrots
3 celery stalks
1 large onion
1 large leek
2-4 large cloves of fresh garlic
2 sprigs fresh oregano leaves
3 bay leaves
4 sprigs fresh thyme
½ bunch parsley
2 tsp ground turmeric
1 tsp cayenne pepper
Pinch of sea salt to taste
2½ quarts cold water

Place all vegetables in a large stockpot cover with cold water. Cook at low heat for 45 minutes-1 hour. Add cayenne pepper, turmeric, and salt and let cook for another 10 minutes. Strain and keep the broth. This will keep in the refrigerator for at least 3 days. **Do not freeze and defrost.** Make fresh as needed.

Juices

Alkalizing juice
3 beet greens (leaves)
4 carrots
½ apple
Handful parsley
Handful spinach
Feed ingredients into juicer one at a time, enjoy immediately!

Liver cleansing juice
1 whole beet
1 celery stalk
3-4 carrots
1 lemon (peeled)
Handful dandelion greens
Feed ingredients into juicer one at a time then enjoy immediately!

Kidney cleansing juice
1 celery stalk
Handful cranberries
Handful parsley
Handful mint leaves
Feed ingredients into juicer one at a time then enjoy immediately!

High calcium juice
Handful spinach
3 kale leaves
Handful parsley
½ green apple
Feed ingredients into juicer one at a time then enjoy immediately!

Protein Powder Shake Recipes

Use: Whey Protein or vegetarian protein (hemp, pea, and/chia combination)

Powder must contain 20-30g protein, <4g carbohydrates with all amino acids profile.

Chocolate mint shake

1 scoop protein powder
1 banana
½ cup fresh mint leaves
1 tsp super foods (spirulina/chlorella/kelp powder)
1 tbsp. chia seeds
1 cup chocolate almond milk
½ cup water
Ice cubes (optional)
Blend all ingredients until smooth in blender and enjoy!

Almond blend

1 scoop protein powder
1 cup spinach
1 small banana
1 tbsp. almond butter
½ tsp almond extract (optional)
½ cup vanilla almond milk
½ cup water
Ice cubes (optional)
Blend all ingredients until smooth in blender and enjoy!

Strawberry morning

1 scoop protein powder
1 cup strawberry
1 tbsp. flax seeds
1 tbsp. chia seeds
1 cup coconut water or almond milk
Ice cubes (optional)
Blend all ingredients until smooth in blender and enjoy!

Energy superfoods
1 scoop protein powder
1 cup blueberries
1 cup spinach or broccoli
1 tsp spirulina powder
1 tsp chlorella powder
1 tsp moringa powder
1 tsp green tea powder
1 tbsp flax seed meal
1 cup green tea
Ice cubes (optional)
Blend all ingredients until smooth and enjoy!

No Protein Powder Smoothies

Green garden smoothie
¼ cup celery
¼ cup fennel
¼ cup spinach
¼ cup frozen peas
1 tbsp. parsley
1 tbsp. lemon juice
Small piece of ginger
2 tbsp. water or almond milk
Ice cubes (optional)
Blend all ingredients until smooth and enjoy!

Tropical smoothie
½ cup papaya
½ cup mango
1 tbsp. lime juice
1 cup coconut water
¼ tsp ground nutmeg or cinnamon
Blend all ingredients until smooth and enjoy!

Green Morning Smoothie
1 cup spinach
1 celery stick
¼ cup goji berries
1 small banana
1 tbsp. almond butter
1 tbsp. chia seeds
1 tsp super foods (spirulina or chlorella)
1 tsp dandelion powder
2 tsp lemon juice
1-2 cups green tea
Ice cubes (optional)
Blend all ingredients until smooth and enjoy!

Red Lunch Smoothie
½ cup pineapple
1 cup kale
1 small beet (chopped)
1 tsp super food (spirulina or chlorella)
1 tbsp. flax seed oil
1 tbsp chia seeds
1 tbsp. lemon juice
1-2 cups coconut water or almond milk
Blend all ingredients in blender and enjoy!

Purple Dinner Smoothie
1 cup avocado
½ cup broccoli
1 cup blueberries
1 cup blackberries
½ cup sprouted almonds
1 tbsp. flax seeds
2 tsp lime juice
1-2 cups coconut water or infused water
Ice cubes (optional)
Blend all ingredients in blender and enjoy!

Breakfast and snack alternatives

Chia seed pudding parfait
3 tbsp. chia seeds
1 cup any liquid (almond milk, water, fresh fruit juice)
1 tbsp. chopped almonds or any other nuts
1-2 strawberries, sliced
¼ cup blueberries
To make chia seed pudding
Add chia seeds to liquid and saturate for 2-4 hours or overnight
To make parfait
Remove pudding from refrigerator (if too thick add more liquid).
Pour into a parfait glass. Add toppings and enjoy!

Perfect Oatmeal
1 cup oats
¼ cup blueberries
¼ cup blackberries
1 tbsp. slivered almond or chopped walnuts
½ cup almond milk
1 cup water
If using quick/instant oats. Boil 1 cup water and add to oats. Let sit for 2-5 minutes then stir in almond milk. Add toppings and enjoy!
For steel oats, option to cook on stovetop or overnight in crockpot at low heat. Then add toppings.

Dressings

Avocado dressing
1 ripe hass avocado
½ tsp dill
¼ tsp sea salt
½ lemon juice or 2 tbsp. lemon juice
½ cup water

Blend all ingredients until smooth.

Vinaigrette
1 part vinegar to 3 parts oil + salt & pepper to taste
Apple cider or Balsamic vinaigrette
1 tbsp. apple cider / balsamic vinegar
3 tbsp. olive oil
½ Lemon juice
Salt & pepper to taste
Whisk until smooth
Add fresh herbs like basil, thyme, dill, or fennel

Light and fresh Salads

Dandelion salad
2 cups dandelion greens
Dressing:
1 garlic clove,
2 tsp lemon juice,
1 tsp olive oil
Sea salt and pepper to taste
Blend ingredients for dressing until smooth
Toss salad with dressing and enjoy!

Shaved Fennel
1 fennel bulb shave thin
2 tbsp. olive oil
2 tbsp. lemon juice
1 twig thyme, chopped
1 tsp parsley
Mix all ingredients and refrigerate for 30minutes. Then serve

Kale salad
2 cups kale (tear)
1 tbsp. fresh lemon juice
2 tsp. apple cider vinegar (optional)

1 tbsp. Braggs liquid aminos
1 tbsp. extra virgin olive oil
Put kale in a bowl and massage lemon juice and vinegar into it. Toss with olive oil and Braggs liquid aminos. Refrigerate for 15-30 minutes then serve. For **chunky kale salad**, add chopped bell peppers, mushrooms, cucumber, Kalamata olives, and tomatoes.

Avocado salad
1 avocado
1 cucumber, diced
1 tomatoes, diced
1 tbsp. fresh finely chopped parsley
½ small red onions, diced
1 tbsp. lemon / lime juice
1 tbsp. olive oil
Cut avocado in half and remove the seed. Spoon the flesh out of the skin. Mash with olive oil and lemon / lime juice. Add remaining ingredients and combine well. Season with salt and pepper. For a refreshing salad, refrigerate before serving.

Colorful Vegetable Slaw
1 cup shredded, peeled broccoli stems
1 cup shredded red cabbage
½ orange bell pepper, cut into thin slivers
1 tbsp. finely chopped parsley
¼ cup olive oil
2 tbsp. fresh lemon juice
Sea salt to taste (1/4 tsp)
Cracked black pepper or cayenne pepper
In a large glass bowl with a lid, mix together broccoli, cabbage, bell pepper, and parsley and set aside. Whisk olive oil, salt, and pepper in a small bowl. Pour dressing on vegetables and toss to combine. Grab lid to cover and refrigerate for 30 min – 1 hour before serving.

Tabbouleh Quinoa Salad
1 cup sprouted quinoa
1 cucumber peeled, seeded, and chopped
1 tomato, chopped
½ red onion chopped
3 tbsp. fresh mint finely chopped
½ cup finely chopped parsley
½ cup olive oil
3 tbsp. lemon juice
Sea salt to taste
In a large bowl combine and mix all ingredients. Cover and refrigerate for 30min - 1 hour.

Side Vegetable Dishes

Hummus
1 cup chickpeas/garbanzo beans
½ cup tahini sauce
1 lemon juice
1-2 garlic cloves
¼ cup olive oil
1 tbsp. ground cumin
Salt & pepper to taste
Add chickpeas to a bowl and rinse. Fill bowl with water and soak peas overnight. Rinse and drain remaining liquid. Cook until soft. In a food processor, combine all ingredients and process until smooth. Add more lemon juice or water to change acidity and consistency as needed.

Cauliflower mashed
½ head cauliflower, chopped
1 tbsp. extra virgin olive oil
Salt and pepper to taste
Steam cauliflower until tender (7-10min). In a food processor, blend cauliflower, olive oil, salt, and pepper until smooth. Transfer to a bowl and enjoy!

Cauliflower rice
½ head cauliflower
1 tbsp olive oil
Salt and pepper to taste other herbs
Grate cauliflower to rice consistency. Blot out extra moisture. Add to warm skillet with olive oil. Season with salt and pepper or fresh herbs. Cook for 5 minutes or until slightly tender.

Grilled asparagus
6 Asparagus spears
1 tbsp. olive or flax seed oil
Sea salt and crack black pepper to taste
Toss asparagus in olive oil, salt, and pepper. Place on grill and grill for 1-2 minutes on each sides. (If using flax seed oil, add oil after grilling). Do not overcook asparagus.

Pea soup
2 tbsp. olive oil
1 shallots (chopped)
2 cloves garlic
½ large leek, trimmed
1 medium potato
1 cup vegetable stock
2 cups fresh or frozen peas
Salt and pepper to taste
Sauté garlic and shallots for 4 min. then add leek and cook for 2 min. Add potatoes (optional) cook for 5 more minutes. Pour in vegetable stock and simmer for 10 minutes until potatoes are cooked. Add in peas, return to boil, and continue to simmer for 2 minutes (if using frozen peas, 10 minutes for fresh peas). Remove from heat, pour into a blender, and blend until completely smooth. Strain, discard the paste, and serve.

Fennel Grilled vegetables
1 crown broccoli
1 bell pepper

1 red onions
1 zucchini
1 tbsp. fennel, chopped
1-2 tbsp. olive oil
½ tsp salt
½ tsp cracked pepper
Combine all ingredients in a bowl. Heat grill and grill vegetables for 3-5 minutes. This will make multiple servings.

Herb Baked Tofu
1 lb. extra firm tofu
1 tbsp. finely chopped fresh basil
1 tbsp. olive oil
1 tbsp. Braggs amino
Whisk basil, olive oil, and soy sauce. Cut tofu into squares and add to mixture. Let marinade for 1 hour. Preheat oven to 400°F. Place tofu on a baking sheet and discard excess liquid. Bake until lightly browned for 7-8 minutes per side. Enjoy! This will make multiple servings.

Poultry Dishes

Roasted Chicken breast
4-6 ounces skinless and boneless chicken breasts
1 tbsp. olive oil
Cayenne or Cracked pepper
Sea salt for flavor
In a Ziploc bag, add chicken breast, olive oil, cracked or cayenne pepper, pinch of sea salt. Mix well in the bag and refrigerate for 1 hour. Preheat oven to 350°F. Roast for 20 min or until juices run clear.

Chicken stir-fry
4-5 oz. chicken breast thinly sliced
1 cup asparagus, chopped
1 cup broccoli, chopped
1 red bell peppers, chopped
1 red onions, chopped
3 tbsp. minced garlic
3 tbsp. minced ginger
4 tbsp. olive oil
Salt and pepper to taste
Combine chicken, 2 tbsp. olive oil, garlic, ginger, salt and pepper in a bowl. Refrigerate for 30min. Heat 2 tbsp. olive oil in a large skillet over medium-high heat. Cook and stir in vegetables until just tender (5 minutes). Remove from heat and set aside. Add chicken into skillet and cook for 2 minutes on each side. Add vegetables and cook for another 5 minutes or until chicken is no longer pink in the middle. Serve.

Rosemary Chicken kabobs
4-6 oz. chicken breast cut into cubes
1 yellow bell pepper
1 red bell pepper
1 small red onion
1 zucchini sliced
1 rosemary twig
4 tbsp. olive oil
Salt and pepper to taste
Soak wooden skewer for 15 minutes in water. Cut chicken breast into cubes and vegetables into 2-inch pieces. In a bowl, combine all ingredients with olive oil. Thread chicken and vegetables alternately onto skewers. Grill for 12-15minutes until chicken juices run clear. Turn frequently. Enjoy!

Lemon Dill Grilled Turkey Breast
4-6 ounces skinless and boneless chicken breasts
2 tbsp. olive oil

1 lemon, juiced
¼ cup freshly chopped dill
Cayenne or Cracked pepper
Sea salt for flavor
In a Ziploc bag, add chicken breast, olive oil, lemon juice, cracked or cayenne pepper, freshly chopped dill, pinch of sea salt. Mix well in the bag and refrigerate for 1 hour. Remove from refrigerator, grill until juices run clear.

Grilled pesto Chicken
4-5oz chicken breast
4 cups fresh basil leaves
½ cup olive oil
2 garlic cloves
1 tsp kosher salt
½ cup pine nuts (optional)
To make pesto, combine all ingredients except chicken and blend until smooth.
In a large Ziploc bag, add chicken breast and pesto. Mix well. Let marinate in the refrigerator for 2 hours or overnight. Heat a grill plate with high heat. Place chicken on grill. Grill until chicken is no longer pink in the middle.

Bunless Turkey Burger
4-6 oz. lean ground turkey breast
2 tsp of freshly chopped parsley
1 tsp olive oil
1 garlic cloves, minced
Salt and cracked black pepper to taste
Mix all ingredients except olive oil until combined. Form burger patty. Heat a small size skillet over medium heat, add olive oil, and cook turkey patty for 4-5 minutes on each side or until liquid is clear. Serve with lettuce, tomatoes, and avocado. (Optional, add cheese in phase II and III only)

Turkey meatballs
4-6 oz. lean ground turkey breast
2 tsp of freshly chopped basil
½ tsp fresh thyme
½ tsp finely chopped rosemary
1 tsp olive oil
1 garlic cloves, minced
Salt and cracked black pepper to taste
Preheat oven to 350°F. Mix all ingredients except olive oil in a bowl until combine. Form turkey into small balls. Heat a small size skillet over medium heat, add olive, and cook turkey meatballs for 4-7 minutes until browned turning occasionally. Place skillet in oven and cook for another 5 minutes. Remove and serve.

Turkey stuffed zucchini
4 zucchini
1 tbsp. olive oil
½ small onion
1 shallot, minced
3 cloves, crushed
½ medium size red bell pepper, diced
1 tsp paprika
1 tsp freshly chopped rosemary
1 tsp freshly chopped basil
Salt & pepper to taste
Preheat oven to 350°F. Cut zucchini in half lengthwise. Using a spoon, scoop out flesh (chop and set aside), leaving a ¼ inch thick. Arrange zucchini in a greased baking dish.
In a saucepan, heat oil then add onions, shallot, and garlic. Cook until onion is transparent. Add chopped zucchini flesh, red bell pepper, and seasoning. Cook for 2-3 minutes. Add ground turkey. Cook until meat is no longer pink.
Spoon into zucchini shells and bake uncovered for 25-30 minutes or until zucchini is tender.

Bunless Portabella burger
2 portabella mushrooms
5 oz. ground buffalo
1 tbsp. olive oil
1 tbsp. butter
¼ cup goat cheese (optional)
1 tbsp. balsamic vinegar
Salt and pepper to taste

To make mushroom
Remove stems from mushroom. With a spoon, scrape the gills from the bottom of the mushroom. In a large skillet over medium heat, melt butter and olive oil. Place mushrooms with the underside down into the pan and cook for about 5 minutes. Flip over, drizzle with balsamic vinegar, season with salt and pepper, and cook for about 4 minutes. Remove and plate.

To make burger
Season meat. Shape into patty. Place onto same skillet. Cook on each side for 4-5minutes. Place burger on mushroom and add lettuce and tomatoes.

Fish and seafood

Grilled dill lemon salmon
1 salmon fillet (3-4oz)
1 lemon
1 tbsp. freshly chopped dill
1tbsp olive oil
1 tsp sea salt
Cracked pepper

In a bowl, combine salmon, ½ lemon juice, olive oil, dill, salt, and pepper. Cover and marinate in refrigerator for 1 hour. Place salmon on heated grill with 2-3 slices of lemon on top. Grill for 3-4 minutes on each side or until salmon is no longer pink in the middle. Do not overcook.

King prawns
4 king prawns (large shrimp)
½ cup olive oil
1 tbsp. Thyme
2 cloves Garlic, minced
1 tsp. Lemon zest
Place prawns in a bowl mix with thyme, garlic, lemon zest, and 1 tbsp. of olive oil. Mix to coat then let marinate in the fridge for 1 hour or overnight.
Heat 2 tbsp. of olive oil in a large saucepan over high heat. Add prawns and sear for 2 minutes, turning once or twice, until they are no longer translucent.

Shrimp wrap
4oz shrimp
½ cup chopped celery
½ cup chopped asparagus
1 garlic clove
1 tsp fresh ginger
1 tbsp. olive
Salt and pepper
2 Romaine lettuce
Heat skillet. Add oil and shrimp. Cook until opaque. Remove from heat and add vegetables to skillet and cook for 2-3minutes. Add cooked shrimp and seasoning. Remove from heat and add to lettuce leaves.

Scallops
3 tbsp. olive oil
Salt and cracked black pepper to taste
½ Lemon juice
Toss scallops with 2 tbsp. olive oil, salt, and cracked black pepper. Place a large frying pan over high heat with 1 tbsp. olive oil. Press scallops down in the pan. Cook for about 2 minutes on each side. Remove from heat and squeeze over the lemon juice.

Seared Tuna
4 oz. tuna
1½ tsp olive oil
¼ tsp salt
1 tbsp. mixed peppercorns
Place in sauté pan on high heat. Sear for 1 min on each side.

Dill Tuna Skewers
3 medium tuna steaks (cut into 1 inch cubes)
1 tbsp. olive oil
1 tbsp. freshly chopped dill
Coarse seal salt and cracked pepper
Mix tuna in a large bowl with dill, olive oil, salt, and pepper. Place 6 cubes of tuna on each skewer and set aside. Place a grill pan over high heat and when hot, add skewer and grill for 3 minutes, turning frequently until all sides are grilled. Serve!

Tips for Long-Term Success

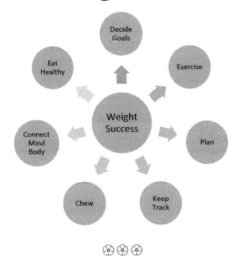

1. Determine your goals

- Decide how much you want to lose and by when

- Determine a start date.

- Create "S.M.A.R.T." goals ("Specific, Measurable, Achievable, Relevant, Time-bound"). For example: I want to lose 10lbs in 30 days by eating healthy, exercising a minimum of 4 days a week, and keeping track of my progress).

- 2-3lbs per week is a reasonable amount of weight to lose without starving yourself or going on crash diets.

- Keep your expectations of yourself reasonable and practical.

- It is extremely important to have a plan of action, a vision, and possibly an accountability partner. (Envisioning your goals create a picture in your mind that begins to make it real).

2. Adapt a healthy diet and lifestyle

- Eat smaller portions –increase metabolism and stabilize blood sugar.

- Avoid second helpings.

- Increase intake of high fiber foods like raw vegetables.

- Avoid overcooking vegetables – lightly steamed, roasted, or sautéed vegetables retain more of their nutritional values than fried or overcooked veggies.

- Include a fair amount of vegetable-source proteins such as beans and bean products (tofu, tempeh), seeds, and nuts for overall health and wellbeing.

- Include Essential Fatty Acids (EFAs) – use cold pressed, and unrefined vegetable oils (e.g., cold water fish, cold pressed flax oil, pumpkin seed oil, walnut oil, and sesame oil)

- Add sea vegetables-seaweeds – nori, wakame, kelp, dulse (high in iodine – increase metabolism).

- Choose organic over non-organic foods. Remember foods grown non-organically often contain pesticides and other chemical residues.

- Eliminate hydrogenated fats: margarine, vegetable shortening, beef and bacon fat, and lard.

- Eat foods in their natural rather than processed form: fresh vegetables vs frozen vegetables vs canned vegetables.

- Restrict refined sugar intake: use honey, maple syrup, fruit juices, agave nectar, and molasses if you must.

- Restrict refined grains such as white rice, white flour products like breads, pasta, and pastries; use whole-grain breads and pasta instead.

- Restrict soda pop and black teas.

- Avoid fried foods, they are high in fat and cholesterol.

- Avoid processed and fast foods, they are usually low in fiber, high in fat, sugar, and salt and contain chemical colorings, flavorings, and preservatives or choose better alternative fast foods.

- **Always Read labels!!!**

- ***Do not eat after 7 PM or 3 hours before your bedtime***

- ***Do not eat starches after 4 pm.***

- **Water: drink a minimum of half your body size in ounces daily.** Follow my rule of 10 during your meals by drinking **10 ounces of water 10 minutes before and 10 minutes after you eat.** More than half of your body is comprised of water, water is very important to weight loss.

- Eat healthy to stay healthy.

3. Chew, Chew, and Chew some more!!!

- Digestion starts in the mouth. Chewing facilitates saliva to mix well with the food and commence the break down process.

- Chewing allows you to savor and taste the nutrients in your food, keeps you full longer, and prevents overeating.

- Chew both liquids and solids.

- Chew a minimum of 22 times before swallowing.

- Chew to maintain a healthy weight.

4. Make exercise part of your daily routine

- Make a commitment to maintain an exercise regimen.

- Start slow and gradual.

- Don't over exert yourself.

- Select exercises you love and enjoy.

- Aim at getting a minimum of 150 minutes of moderate-intensity or 75 minutes of vigorous-intensity aerobic exercise, at least two strength-training activities per week, core and flexibility training three times per week.

- Follow the exercises outlined in the exercise training program.
- Check with your physician before beginning any exercise regimen especially if you have any chronic health issues.

5. Connect the mind with the body
- Foster a positive attitude
- Remain patient with your progress.
- See yourself where you would like to be.
- Allow your mind to believe that your body can achieve your weight loss goals.

6. Plan, Plan, Plan!!!

- Planning leads to success.
- Plan your meals at the beginning of the week and begin to make preparation steps.
- Make your grocery list and be ready to go shopping on Sunday.
- Plan to eat healthy snacks between meals (protein shake in between or dividing your 3 heavy meals into 6 smaller meals).
- ***Do not starve yourself!!!***
- Factor in exercise in your daily routine. Wake up a little earlier to include cardio before your first meal and strength training before or after your last meal.

♦ Schedule time to journal and meditate.

7. Keep track

♦ Studies have shown that people who keep track of their daily diet and exercise routine by recording them on paper or electronic devices are more successful at achieving long-term weight loss goals than those who do not.

♦ Keep a daily record of your food intake and your exercise routine.

♦ Keep track of foods that produce allergic responses, increase body weight and blood pressure, spike blood sugar, and cause inflammation then remove them out of the diet.

♦ Write your weekly plans and goals for the week and daily affirmations.

♦ Purchase a pedometer to stay on track.

With determination, a plan, a vision, self-appreciation, love, proper diet and exercise, and self-discipline you can achieve just about anything. You will begin to develop new patterns of eating while taking care of yourself and your needs. You have all the tools to assist you along the way and keep you well and healthy beyond the program.

Stay well, be well, and believe in yourself!!!

HE + E + MBC = R4S

53796949R00135

Made in the USA
Lexington, KY
19 July 2016